Red Flags: A Guide to Identifying Serious Pathology of the Spine

For Elsevier:

Publisher Heidi Harrison
Development Editor Siobhan Campbell
Project Manager Emma Riley
Design Andrew Chapman
Illustrator Jonathan Haste
Illustration Buyer Gillian Murray

Red Flags:
A Guide to Identifying Serious Pathology of the Spine

Sue Greenhalgh MA GD Phys MCSP

Consultant Physiotherapist, Bolton PCT, Bolton, UK

James Selfe PhD MA GD Phys MCSP

Professor in Physiotherapy, University of Central Lancashire, Preston, UK

Foreword by

Louis Gifford MAppSc BSc FCSP

Chartered Physiotherapist, Falmouth Physiotherapy Clinic, Cornwall, UK

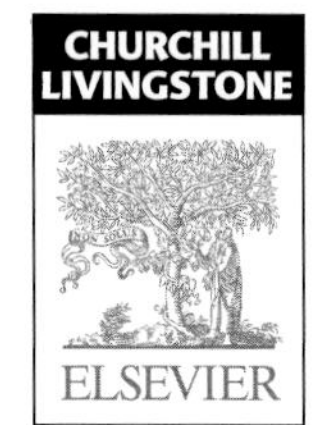

EDINBURGH LONDON NEW YORK OXFORD
PHILADELPHIA ST LOUIS SYDNEY TORONTO
2006

CHURCHILL
LIVINGSTONE
ELSEVIER

An imprint of Elsevier Limited

First published 2006
Reprinted 2007, 2009

ISBN 978 0 4431 0140 3

British Library Cataloguing in Publication Data
A catalogue record for this book is available from the British Library.

Library of Congress Cataloging in Publication Data
A catalog record for this book is available from the Library of Congress.

Note
Neither the Publisher nor the Authors assume any responsibility for any loss or injury and/or damage to persons or property arising out of or related to any use of the material contained in this book. It is the responsibility of the treating practitioner, relying on independent expertise and knowledge of the patient, to determine the best treatment and method of application for the patient.

Printed in China

The Publisher's policy is to use paper manufactured from sustainable forests.

Contents

Foreword

I have always believed that every patient who goes to see their doctor wants to know the following:

- Doctor, what's wrong with me?
- Doctor, how long is it going to take to get better?
- Doctor, is there anything that I can do to help it get better?
- Doctor, is there anything that you can do or give me to help it?

The order of importance to each individual may alter slightly, but for most, a reassuring answer to the first question is always somewhere near the top. Implicit here is a simple desire to know whether there is something seriously wrong. It is often the most important starting point for a successful treatment outcome.

Perhaps clinicians need to think about this more, because without a thorough understanding and without reassurance, the patient's progress is likely to be hampered by feelings of uncertainty and insecurity. Would you go back to work, comply with a series of exercises or take a prescribed medicine if you still had an uneasy inkling that something was badly wrong or something had been missed?

A great many patients, acute and chronic, report that they have not been listened to fully, not examined fully and not been reassured or had an adequate explanation of their symptoms. Many people with benign pain complaints remain burdened by uncertainty and hence are unable to recover in any meaningful way. The title of an old but very important article by Nortin Hadler always rings in my ears: 'If you have to prove you are ill, you can't get well' (Hadler 1996). The main message for me is: 'Top-down before bottom-up', which simply means that for every clinical encounter undertaken it is the clinician's responsibility to reassure the patient (top-down), before embarking on the 'physical' (bottom-up) recovery pathway.

In my daily dealings with patients I frequently hear about pain that comes on for no reason and often quite severely, about pain that keeps the patient awake at night, that gets rapidly worse and pain that the patient thinks is something serious. Patients are naturally worried; after all, worry is what often drives their help-seeking behaviour.

I strongly believe that in order to be successful all good therapists need to be far more explicit here. At the end of every first session with all my patients I state/ask the following: 'It is important before moving on with treatment/rehabilitation that you feel comfortable that I have listened to all your problems, all your concerns and examined you fully. I need you to feel reassured about what is wrong and the recovery process. Do you have any concerns?'.

You simply cannot ask this question if you are not confident, if you do not know.

Having up-to-date 'Red Flag' knowledge is essential for clinician confidence and in turn for patient confidence – every therapist or doctor should be able to say to every patient seen that they been through a check list of features that signifies a serious disorder and the need for further investigation.

This book is so important and so timely as we start to learn more and more about the importance of clinician–patient interactions. Reassurance is a pain killer, and you cannot give reassurance if you are unsure!

This is a book that every clinician should have a personal copy of and continue to refer to throughout their whole professional life.

Louis Gifford

Reference

Hadler N M 1996 If you have to prove you are ill, you can't get well. The object lesson of fibromyalgia. Spine 21(20): 2397–2400

Acknowledgements

We would like to thank Guy McLennan for his typing skills and good humour.

We would also like to thank Louis Gifford and Steve Young for their constructive criticism and support.

Introduction

The Chartered Society of Physiotherapy describes 1978 as a 'watershed' in the physiotherapy profession. It was in this year that physiotherapists became clinically autonomous in the UK. Today access to physiotherapy is still largely controlled by a traditional medical model. However, these are changing times with modernization, blurring of professional boundaries and more creative ways of delivering healthcare. Physiotherapists are coming increasingly into the spotlight at the cutting edge of healthcare provision. There is widening access to physiotherapy by innovations such as telephone help lines, increased patient choice and improved timing of care. This book has been written for musculoskeletal physiotherapists, students, lecturers and other practitioners who work with patients complaining of spinal pain. Six out of ten people will feel back pain at some time in their life, many seeking medical help; 1% of these cases will have serious pathology. These changing times, inevitably, put clinicians in a position where they will be faced with serious spinal pathology. This book is devoted in its entirety to helping to identify the 1% of cases with:

- tumour
- infection or
- other conditions requiring urgent specialist investigation and treatment (e.g. fractures).

Grieve (1994) suggests that the identification of serious pathology depends more on 'awareness, vigilance and suspicion rather than a set of rules'. This book endeavours to provide a set of guidelines to raise awareness and vigilance and provoke appropriate suspicion. Gifford & Butler (1997) suggest that clinical reasoning is an analytical process in which data from a variety of sources, pertinent to the patient's unique clinical scenario, are examined. This book contains a valuable range of data to support this reasoning process with respect to serious spinal pathology.

We will endeavour to answer your questions about indicators for serious pathology (Red Flags) that we have been frequently asked. The answers are often embedded in a diverse literature and difficult to find. This book consolidates these facts into a concise, readable summation of important Red Flag details. In addition, it provides a sounder, more robust basis on which to make a clinical decision by providing an 'index of suspicion' cutting through the 'red haze' surrounding Red Flags. The index of suspicion for each Red Flag item is denoted by an attached flag system – those with a higher index have a larger number of flags. It clarifies issues such as:

- How much weight loss is considered significant?
- Is the risk of developing serious pathology the same at 6 years, 16 years and 66 years of age?

We explore and discuss a number of terms including three-dimensional thinking, conditional probabilities and 'Red Herrings'. The term Red Herring originates from the very pungent salted and smoked herrings, which were red in colour, used by anti-hunting campaigners in the 1800s to create false trails. The hounds invariably followed the false trails created by these Red Herrings, allowing the fox to escape. In this book we use the term Red Herrings in a broad way as a concept that incorporates psychosocial and biomedical parameters. Red Herrings are an important phenomenon to be aware of as they can mislead the clinician and confuse the clinical picture, leading to unnecessary and sometimes catastrophic delay in ultimate diagnosis.

We hope that you are as excited as we are by the possibilities that this book creates. We consider that our 'index of suspicion' can be a vital tool in the clinical decision-making process. By weighting Red Flags, critical conditions can be more rapidly identified. The contents of this book will boost confidence in your own clinical judgement by helping you to collate the appropriate information and logically process these findings. If serious pathology is identified at an early stage, clinicians can raise the alarm to potentially greatly improve a patient's prognosis. This will ultimately add to your own empowerment and rewards within your role. The technical application of physiotherapy is relatively straightforward. The challenge lies partly in knowing which techniques to apply to which patients but above all in not only knowing when physiotherapy is inappropriate but recognizing when something serious is going on.

References

Grieve G P 1994 The masqueraders. In: Boyling J D, Palastanga N (eds) Grieve's modern manual therapy: the vertebral column, 2nd edn. Churchill Livingstone, Edinburgh, p 841–856

Gifford L, Butler D S 1997 The integration of pain sciences into clinical practice. Journal of Hand Therapy 10:86–95

Chapter 1

Red Flags

CHAPTER CONTENTS

In recent years there has been an increased demand for musculoskeletal medicine. This has led to a dramatic expansion in a number of professions involved in the management of musculoskeletal disorders. For example, across the European Union the number of physiotherapists increased by 21% between 1996 and 1999 (European Commission 2004). Along with these changes, healthcare systems are evolving and being reorganized. In the European Union there has been a major shift towards managing patients in primary care with a result that the number of acute hospital beds fell by 30% between 1980 and 2000 (European Commission 2004).

Simultaneous to these developments physiotherapists have expanded their role and are more commonly taking on the role of first contact and extended scope practitioners in a variety of non-traditional settings. These changes in practice are leading to challenges and opportunities not previously faced by the physiotherapy profession. Many of the conditions we discuss in this book have been around for centuries. However, more physiotherapists are now increasingly likely to come into contact with these serious cases earlier in the disease processes where previously they may not have seen them at all.

In the United Kingdom the Chartered Society of Physiotherapy (CSP) has established a clinical interest group dedicated to extended scope practitioners (ESPs). The membership stood at 250 in 2004 (CSP 2004). The role of extended scope physiotherapy practitioners includes:

- requesting investigations, e.g. blood tests, scans, X-rays, nerve conduction studies
- using the result of investigations to assist clinical diagnosis and appropriate management of patients
- listing for surgery
- referring to other medical and paramedical professions.

It is difficult to determine exactly how many patients with serious spinal pathology present to physiotherapists. During a 7-year period of working in a specialist spinal assessment clinic where 1000 patients were seen annually, it is estimated by one of the authors that on average there was 1 patient a month who presented with serious spinal pathology of some type. In comparison, it is reported that an average general practitioner in England or Wales will see approximately 8 or 9 new cases of cancer each year (Department of Health 2000a). It is therefore important that physiotherapists remain vigilant to the possibility that the patient in front of them may have a serious pathology.

HISTORICAL PERSPECTIVE OF PHYSIOTHERAPY

According to Cyriax (1982), the first mention of a professor of physiotherapy dates from AD 585. Rehabilitation in ancient Greece and Rome was described by Hippocrates and other scholars. At around the time that Daniel David Palmer was founding chiropractic in North America, the London massage scandal of

1894 galvanized legislators in Britain to regulate masseuses. The profession had fallen into disrepute and massage parlours were being described by the *British Medical Journal* as hotbeds of vice (Barclay 1994). In 1894 Miss Rosalind Paget and Miss Lucy Robinson, two qualified masseuses, took steps to redeem the reputation of massage as a respectable treatment. This eventually led to the birth of the Chartered Society of Physiotherapy. In 1973, in the UK, the McMillan report moved the physiotherapy profession forwards dramatically by recommending professional autonomy allowing physiotherapists greater responsibility and freedom to treat and diagnose (Barclay 1994). Development of professional autonomy has continued to now include extended scope practitioner and consultant physiotherapist posts (Department of Health 2000b).

EARLY DEVELOPMENT OF INDICATORS OF SERIOUS PATHOLOGY

Historically the profession of physiotherapy has relied on the medical profession for recognition. According to Roberts (1994), the founders of the Chartered Society of Physiotherapy 'traded professional autonomy for the respectability offered by doctors'. The relationship has often been paternalistic on the part of medicine towards physiotherapy. Under these conditions physiotherapists often took the role of technicians carrying out treatments that were prescribed by doctors. However, in their teaching early modern day medical advocates of manual therapy, such as James Mennell and James

Cyriax, not only embraced the profession of physiotherapy but recognized the potential for, and started to encourage, independent practice.

Mennell was actively influencing physiotherapy training as early as the First World War (Barclay 1994). In the introduction of his classic book *The Science and Art of Joint Manipulation* he implies that for doctors to prescribe only one treatment restricts the potential of a successful outcome of physiotherapy (Mennell 1949).

Cyriax describes devoting his whole life to perfecting a method of clinical examination which led to accurate diagnosis of locomotor disorders. His medical peers considered him to be something of a maverick as not only did he develop manipulation techniques which he practised himself but he also taught these diagnostic and treatment techniques to physiotherapists (Cyriax 1982).

Within their teaching both Mennell and Cyriax were aware of the need for caution in some presentations. However, unlike their historical predecessors Mennell and Cyriax both realized that the indication of serious pathology could be more subtle than waiting for its obvious visible manifestation. This prompted them to highlight certain presentations which could suggest something sinister as the underlying cause.

Mennell's Red Flags (Mennell 1952)

- Smallpox
- Influenza
- Genitourinary (gonorrhoea)
- Prostate cancer
- Acute kidney problems
- Multiple sclerosis
- Parkinson's disease
- Tuberculosis (TB)
- Paget's disease
- Appendicitis
- Sepsis – bowel/teeth/tonsillitis
- Haemorrhoids

Cyriax's Red Flags (Cyriax 1982)

- Backache with fever
- Neoplasm
- Root pain >8 months' duration or with gross limitation of every movement
- Weak psoas major
- Afebrile osteomyelitis
- Aortic occlusion
- Spinal claudication
- Nutritional osteomalacia
- Gonorrhoeal fasciitis
- Multiple root palsy
- 'Forbidden area' (thoracolumbar junction pain, should be considered suspiciously)

One of the problems with the way these conditions are presented is that unfortunately they are incorporated into different parts of the main body of the text; extensive reading is therefore necessary before clinicians can access these important facts.

It is also important to consider the major influence of the work of physiotherapists Robin McKenzie and Geoffrey Maitland on the field of musculoskeletal medicine. It is interesting to see how McKenzie's attitude towards the identification of Red Flags appears to have evolved. In the 1990 edition of his book on the cervical and thoracic spine, McKenzie (1990) states: 'It has always been my belief that the differential diagnosis should be established by the patient's family practitioner . . . The patient once screened by the medical practitioner, should have had unsuitable pathologies excluded.' However, in McKenzie's latest edition of his lumbar spine book (McKenzie & May 2003) there is a chapter on serious spinal pathology that discusses some of the Red Flags; in this chapter it is stated: 'serious spinal conditions . . . need early identification and onward referral'. This implies that there is now a role for physiotherapists in recognizing serious pathology.

The most recent edition of *Maitland's Vertebral Manipulation* includes a chapter titled 'The doctor's role in diagnosis and prescribing vertebral manipulation' (Brewerton 2001). This implies that doctors retain the role of initially recognizing serious pathology; in the UK this is not now always the case. However, it is true that historically physiotherapy has relied on the medical profession to provide an accurate diagnosis of the patient's condition which would then inform the physiotherapist's decision to treat. Whilst Maitland states that malignancy of the vertebral column is a contraindication to manual techniques, no guidance for identifying indicators of serious conditions is given.

The current teaching on Red Flags within orthopaedic medicine (Ombregt et al 2003) is more specific; the following warning signs in the subjective history of the cervical spine are described:

- gradual increase in pain; prolonged timescale compared to discogenic patterns
- expanding pain, i.e. spreading across a number of segments rather than shifting within a segment
- bilateral arm pain: suggests non-discal lesion
- radicular pain below 35 years of age
- arm pain over 6 months' duration
- elderly patient with initial presentation or rapid increase in pain or stiffness over 1 or 2 months
- arm pain increased by cough
- paraesthesia all over body provoked by neck flexion
- cord symptoms
- dysphagia
- progressive neck pain at night
- history of cancer.

In addition, the following warning signs in the objective examination of the cervical spine are listed:

Articular

- Painful restriction in full articular pattern in short period of time
- Gross limitation of rotations
- End feel soggy, empty or muscle spasm
- Side flexion away: only painful movement
- Scapular elevation limited.

Non-articular

- Unusual myotome involvement:
  - T1 palsy
  - excessive loss of power
  - two or three nerve root signs and symptoms
  - painless weakness
  - resisted movements of neck not only painful but weak
- Distal symptoms before central
- Anaemia
- Horner's syndrome
- Hoarse voice.

Whilst this teaching is very specific there is now a wealth of information but no apparent system of weighting given to different symptoms and signs. For example, how important is hoarse voice in isolation in someone who has a cervical spine problem? This may cause inappropriate levels of distress if clinical reasoning processes do not consider the overall picture and the conditional probabilities (see Ch. 2).

Apart from the development of Red Flag lists within specific schools of thought, there have also been significant developments in government-driven initiatives. These have attempted to collate a wide range of research-based data and present evidence-based guidelines in user-friendly formats.

CLINICAL GUIDELINES

Over the past three decades there has been a well-recognized increase in the levels of disability associated with spinal problems, with leading authorities referring to back pain as 'a 20th century medical disaster' (Waddell 2004). This has occurred despite the plethora of publications in relation to the management of back pain. However, there have been significant positive developments in the form of clinical guidelines for the diagnosis and management of spinal pain.

Quebec Task Force report 1987

The first of these guidelines was the Quebec Task Force report (Spitzer 1987). This was commissioned as a consequence of an increase in debilitating back pain in the working population of Quebec, Canada. The Task Force was particularly concerned with work status.

In addition, the report described 11 diagnostic categories for spinal disorders.

Quebec Task Force diagnostic categories (Spitzer 1987)

- Pain without radiation
- Pain and radiation to extremity above knee or elbow
- Pain and radiation to extremity below knee or elbow
- Pain and radiation into limb with neurological signs
- Presumptive compression of a spinal nerve root on a simple roentgenogram (i.e. spinal instability or fracture)
- Compression of a spinal nerve root confirmed by specific imaging techniques
- Spinal stenosis
- Post-surgical status 1–6 months
- Post-surgical status >6 months intervention (asymptomatic/symptomatic)
- Chronic pain syndrome
- Other diagnosis

It is interesting to note when reviewing this list that serious pathology would be classified under the vague diagnostic category of 'Other diagnosis'.

Incorporated within the main body of the text the following indicators suggest that more serious disease may be present:

- age <20 or >50 years
- history and/or signs of serious trauma
- history of neoplasm
- fever
- neurological deficit.

The report suggests 'Upon identifying such clinical indicators the clinician should order appropriate paraclinical tests (e.g. plain roentgenograms of the spine, inflammatory or osseous laboratory evaluation, myelography, CT scan or radionucleotide bone scan)'.

CSAG report 1994

In the United Kingdom in 1991 the Clinical Standards Advisory Group (CSAG) was set up as an independent source of expert advice to the Ministry of Health. It was commissioned 'to advise on standards of clinical care for, and access to and availability of services to NHS patients with back pain' (CSAG 1994). CSAG considered duration of back pain and work loss as significant predictors of outcome. It was reported that 90% of low back pain recovered spontaneously in the first 6 weeks. However, if work loss continued for more than 6 months there was only a 50% chance of sufferers returning to their original employment. This report appears to be the first to use the phrase 'Red Flags' for describing diagnostic indicators of serious spinal pathology.

Five diagnostic categories for spinal disorders (CSAG 1994)

- Simple backache
- Nerve root pain
- Red Flags
- Cauda equina syndrome/widespread neurological disorder
- Inflammatory disorder

CSAG goes on to describe the diagnostic triage. This highlights the clinical importance of assessing that patients have musculoskeletal problems. Non-spinal and serious pathologies should be excluded from the diagnosis and the presence and extent of any nerve root pathology determined.

Diagnostic triage CSAG (1994)

- Simple backache (95% of cases)
- Nerve root pain (<5% of cases)
- Possible serious spinal pathology (<1% of cases)

Historically medical triage involves the screening of patients into three priority groups. It developed in response to the problem of dealing with large numbers of wartime casualties:

- those who will die despite intervention (no treatment given)
- those who will survive without intervention (no treatment given)
- those who will only survive with intervention (treatment given).

Triage in back pain applies exactly the same principle, when the following conditions are suspected:

- simple mechanical low back pain (medical intervention not appropriate)

- nerve root pain (in a small proportion medical intervention necessary)
- serious pathology (medical intervention essential) (Gifford 2000).

Red Flags are described as indicators of possible serious spinal pathology. They are physical risk factors of significant medical pathology (Kendall et al 1997). It is important to recognize that the Red Flags represent an interesting list of clinical findings rather than diagnostic labels. This list equips physiotherapists further to fulfil their expanding and extended role in the management of musculoskeletal disorders and as such helps facilitate a paradigm shift for the profession.

Red Flags (CSAG 1994)

- Age of onset <20 or >55 years
- Violent trauma, e.g. fall from a height, road traffic accident
- Constant progressive, non-mechanical pain
- Thoracic pain
- Past medical history of carcinoma
- Systemic steroids
- Drug abuse, HIV
- Systemically unwell
- Weight loss
- Persistent severe restriction of lumbar flexion
- Widespread neurology
- Structural deformity

AHCPR guidelines 1994

Also published in 1994 was the United States Agency for Health Care Policy and Research (AHCPR) clinical guide for the assessment and treatment of acute low back problems in adults (Bigos 1994). The aims of the AHCPR guide were to help patients improve their activity tolerance and to 'provide information on the detection of serious conditions that occasionally cause low back symptoms'.

Similar to the CSAG report the AHCPR guidelines describe diagnostic categories and a list of Red Flags.

AHCPR diagnostic categories (Bigos 1994)

- Potentially serious spinal condition
- Sciatica
- Non-specific back symptoms

A comparison between the AHCPR and CSAG lists of Red Flags shows that both lists are virtually identical; there are three main differences between the two lists. AHCPR includes:

- age of onset >50 rather than >55
- pain that worsens when supine
- severe night-time pain.

It is interesting to note that the AHCPR guidelines like the Quebec Task Force report suggest a more conservative upper limit for age of onset, i.e. 50 years compared to 55 years in the CSAG report.

More recently the Royal College of General Practitioners (2001), the New Zealand Acute Low Back Pain Guide (New Zealand Ministry of Health 2004), and the European guidelines for prevention in low back pain (European Union 2004) have provided back pain guidelines. However, no significant additions to those Red Flags listed in previous publications have emerged.

RED HERRINGS AND MASQUERADERS

We introduced the term Red Herrings in the paper 'Margaret: a tragic case of spinal Red Flags and Red Herrings' (Greenhalgh & Selfe 2004). We consider the term to be broad and to encompass any misleading biomedical or psychosocial factors that will deflect the course of accurate clinical reasoning. Grieve (1994) and Boissonnault (1995) both highlight the importance of differential biomedical diagnosis in the clinical examination of spinal pain.

Grieve describes in some detail misleading presentations of spinal pain; he suggests that virtually any pathology in the abdomen can present with back pain, for example peptic ulcer, cancer of the colon, rectum, pancreas or aortic aneurysm. Not surprisingly there is overlap between the CSAG list and these pathologies, for example:

- gallbladder – only refers pain to thoracic spine region
- multiple myeloma – peak incidence 60–70 years
- tight filum terminale – peak incidence 12–16 years
- the majority of secondary tumours occur above 50 years
- angina – posterior thoracic pain.

Grieve points out that simple thoracic dysfunction can frequently mimic the pain of angina. Similarly thoracic pain can be produced by:

- aorta
- lungs
- oesophagus
- diaphragm
- stomach and duodenum
- liver, gallbladder and bile duct
- pancreas
- spleen
- small intestine, appendix and colon
- kidneys
- reproductive system (Ombregt et al 2003).

Another common symptom that may be benign or that may have serious underlying causes is headache. Physiotherapists commonly see cases of headache that is musculoskeletal in origin; however, Grieve (1994) discusses the differential symptoms of headache due to brain tumour.

Differential symptoms of headache due to brain tumour (Grieve 1994)

- Deep dull constant ache
- Aggravated by being upright
- Not rhythmic or throbbing
- Sometimes severe
- Usually relieved by aspirin or cold packs
- Does not usually disturb sleep
- Aggravated by coughing, sneezing, straining
- Nausea not common
- May be associated with cervical dysfunction

Boissonnault (1995) adopts a systems approach and guides clinicians through each of the body's major systems and highlights questions which may help identify pathologies arising from those systems.

Key signs and symptoms for the cardiovascular system are:

- pain: angina or in legs
- sweating
- palpitations
- breathlessness/cough
- light-headedness/loss of consciousness
- fatigue (Boissonnault 1995).

Tables 1.1 and 1.2 show the main areas of pain referral from the male and female urogenital systems.

TABLE 1.1 REFERRED PAIN: MALE UROGENITAL SYSTEM (BOISSONNAULT 1995)

Structure	Segmental innervation	Possible areas of pain referral
Kidney	T10–L1	Lumbar spine, (ipsilateral) flank Upper abdominal
Ureter	T11–L2, S2–S4	Groin, upper/lower abdominal, suprapubic, scrotum, medial proximal thigh Thoracolumbar
Urinary bladder	T11–L2, S2–S4	Sacral apex, suprapubic Thoracolumbar
Prostate gland	T11–L1, S2–S4	Sacral, low lumbar, testes Thoracolumbar
Testes	T10–T11	Lower abdominal, sacral

Grieve (1994) and Boissonnault (1995) both give very specific and detailed descriptions of certain pathologies, whereas the various Red Flag lists provide clinicians with a more general toolbox of indictors suggesting that something more serious may be occurring. Grieve suggests that recognition of pathology early depends on

TABLE 1.2 REFERRED PAIN: FEMALE UROGENITAL SYSTEM (BOISSONNAULT 1995)

Structure	Segmental innervation	Possible areas of pain referral
Ovaries	T10–T11	Lower abdomen, low back
Uterus	T10–L1	Lower abdomen, low back
Fallopian tubes	T10–L1	Lower abdomen, low back
Perineum	S2–S4	Sacral apex, suprapubic, rectum
External genitalia	L1–L2, S3–S4	Lower abdomen, medial anterior thigh, sacrum
Kidney	T10–L1	Ipsilateral low back and upper abdominal
Urinary bladder	T11–L2, S2–S4	Thoracolumbar, sacrococcygeal, suprapubic
Ureters	T11–L2, S2–S4	Groin, upper and lower abdomen, suprapubic, anterior-medial thigh, thoracolumbar

awareness, vigilance and suspicion rather than rules. One of the potential problems facing clinicians is an overreliance on the Red Flag list. It is important to remember that the Red Flag lists are lists of clinical indicators rather than absolute rules. For example, when considering the age of patients in most clinical practice, age over 50 years on its own should not raise an alarm but should instil a sense of awareness in the physiotherapist's mind.

SOME PATHOLOGIES APPEARING ON RED FLAG LISTS

One of the interesting things that has emerged during our brief historical review is that threats to public health (including spinal dysfunction) are subject to change through time and vary from place to place and that these can influence behaviour in society. In Victorian Britain life for the majority of the population was short and harsh; for example, a 21-year-old labourer could only expect to live to the age of 50 (Thackray Museum 2004). Infectious diseases like tuberculosis (TB) spread rapidly due to poor living conditions. It was not until the mid 19th century that there was recognition of the link between poverty and poor health (McGrew 1985). It is important that clinicians today are aware of these changes and adapt to a changing world. Physiotherapy training only 20 years ago would not have considered conditions such as HIV/AIDS, MRSA or BSE/CJD.

Cancer

Cancer is the term used to define any condition arising from the uncontrolled division and multiplication of cells. There are two basic types of tumour, benign or malignant. A benign tumour will remain localized whereas a malignant tumour will spread (metastasize). Over 100 different cancers have been identified; they can affect any part of the body. The American Cancer Society considers 5% of cancer to be genetic and 95% associated with other confounding factors. Approximately one-third of the population will suffer a form of invasive cancer in their lifetime (Goodman et al 1998).

Evidence of tumours has been recorded across many centuries. Tumours in dinosaurs from the Cretaceous age have been found. Egyptian mummies from the 3rd to 5th dynasties (3000–2500 BC) also displayed evidence of neoplasms; there have also been similar findings in Inca remains (McGrew 1985). The Edwin Smith papyrus (1660 BC) discusses the 'bulging tumour of the breast' for which there was no cure (McGrew 1985). Early medical diagnosis of cancer relied on the visible manifestation of the disease. Hippocrates was the first to coin the term cancer and discussed a variety of descriptive terms including 'karkinoma' or 'karkinos'. After the 6th century AD cancer is frequently discussed in the European medical literature (McGrew 1985).

In the late 16th century a professor of medicine at Basel, post autopsy, described a brain tumour in a knight who had demonstrated bizarre behaviour for 2 years preceding his death (McGrew 1985). Soot was one of the earliest carcinogenic agents to be identified, producing a high incidence of cancer of the scrotum among 18th century chimney sweeps. In the 18th century cancer was considered to develop as a consequence of inflammation (McGrew 1985).

It was not until the early 19th century that Marie François Xavier Bichat, a young French anatomist, discovered that cancers were not inflammations but an overgrowth of cells. In the 19th and 20th centuries it was seen that people working with X-rays, radium or radioactive material had a high cancer rate. Other causes identified were smoking, nutritional deficiencies, alcohol abuse and over-exposure to direct sunlight. The early 20th century saw a rise in the general awareness of cancer (McGrew 1985).

Cancer causes 6 million deaths every year; this is 12% of all deaths worldwide (WHO 2004a). Cancer is predominantly a modern disease associated with increasing lifespan. Across the European Union life expectancy has increased in all countries since 1960; it is currently estimated that 16.2% of the population of Europe is now over 64 years of age. It is also estimated both in Europe and in Australia that 1 in 3 males and 1 in 4 females will develop cancer by the age of 75 (European Commission 2004, Australian Department of Health and Ageing 2004). The World Health Organization (WHO) states that 10 million people are diagnosed with cancer every year and predict that there will be 15 million new cases every year by 2020 (WHO 2004a). Success in controlling other diseases, along with modern environmental dangers inherent in technologically sophisticated civilizations, has also contributed to the rise in cancer. Types of cancer vary geographically; for example, colon cancer is more common in urban areas and skin cancer more common among farmers in rural areas. Interestingly, genetic and chromosomal cancers caused by the environment, e.g. chemical radiation, can pass to the next generation. Recent studies relate cancer to stress. Long-term stress can cause hormonal or immunological changes; this can promote the development of cancer cells. Psychological depression or anxiety can lead to a poorer repair of damaged DNA and changes in apoptosis (cell death) (Goodman et al 1998).

Cancer risk factors (Goodman et al 1998)

- Age
- Lifestyle
    - Tobacco
    - Alcohol
    - Diet
    - Sexual
- Viral
- Geographical
- Environmental
- Gender
- Ethnicity
- Socioeconomic
- Occupation
- Genetics
- Precancerous lesions
- Stress

Commonest cancers worldwide (WHO 2004a)

- Lung – men
- Stomach – men
- Breast – women
- Cervical – women

Lung cancer is the largest group of cancers related to death in both genders (Goodman et al 1998). Current medical practice attempts to identify cancer at the earliest possible stage, even before symptoms arise (Table 1.3). Once symptoms of cancer have developed the outcome is inevitably worse.

Stages of cancer development (Pfalzer 1995)

Precancerous
- Hypertrophy
- Neoplastic hyperplasia (increased number of cells)
- Dysplasia (replacement of mature cells with immature cells)
- Metaplasia (replacement of mature cells with cells of a different type)
- Anaplasia (cellular disorganization)

Cancerous (neoplasia – non-random autonomous cell growth)
- Invasion
- Metastatic process

Escape of malignant cells from immune surveillance

TABLE 1.3 EARLY DETECTION OF ASYMPTOMATIC CANCER (GOODMAN ET AL 1998)

	Risk factors	Test
Breast	Women >40 years	Breast examination Annual mammogram
Uterus	All sexually active women	Pap test Pelvic examination
Endometrium	Hereditary	Endometrial biopsy >35 years
Prostate	>50 years African/American History in first degree relative	Prostate specific PSA blood test Digital rectal examination

The spread of cancer can be speeded up by ageing, a dysfunctional immune system, hormonal and environmental changes, pregnancy and stress (Goodman et al 1998). Metastases are believed to pass from primary sites as emboli into the venous system; these pass via the heart and lungs to reach the vertebral bodies as arterial emboli. It is estimated that between 50% and 70% of patients with cancer develop metastases before death. This figure can be as high as 85% for women with breast cancer (Wiesel et al 1996). Metastases and primary tumours occur at all sites in the spine and at any age (Wiesel et al 1996). Cervical primary tumours account for 4.2% of all primary bone tumours; both primary tumours and metastases present much less frequently in the cervical spine than in the thoracic or lumbar spines (Ombregt et al 2003).

The high incidence of secondary metastases in the vertebral bodies, ribs and ilium is most probably explained by the slower bloodstream at these haemopoietic sites in the adult (Grieve 1981). Malignancy affects the vertebral body four times more frequently than the posterior spinal elements. To be visible on X-ray 30–50% destruction of the vertebral body needs to have occurred. Although the vertebral body is the area most commonly affected at initial presentation, it is often pedicle destruction that is observed initially by X-ray; here minimal changes can be observed on X-ray (Wiesel et al 1996). The goal of treatment in cases of spinal metastases is generally palliative as treatment is seldom curative (Ratliff & Cooper 2004).

Metastases often present 2–5 years after initial diagnosis. Low grade lesions, however, can develop metastases as much as 20 years later (Goodman et al 1998). Grieve also suggests that the position of neoplastic disease in relation to the caudal or cephalad site affects prognosis. He suggests that the more cranial the lesion the poorer the outcome (Grieve 1981). Cancers that spread to bone first have a poorer prognosis (Goodman et al 1998).

Survival times vary with spinal metastases of different origin (Ratliff & Cooper 2004). With cancer of the colon, median survival time is less than 3 months; for melanoma it is 4 months.

Other factors contributing to the spread of metastases include speed of onset, length of symptoms and sphincter involvement. Secondaries spread more rapidly in younger patients and metastases from the lungs are much more aggressive than those from breast, prostate, thyroid or kidney (Grieve 1994). Metastases often possess the same cellular structure as that of the primary growth and this can enable the primary to be identified (Goodman et al 1998).

It is particularly interesting to note that pelvic tumours were found to take an average of 61 weeks to diagnosis due to the low level of suspicion aroused in clinicians (Table 1.4). Thirteen out of seventy cases went on to have negative initial radiograph results although evidence of serious pathology was seen on retrospective review (Grieve 1994). There are two main technical difficulties in detecting pelvic tumours. The first relates to the standard view used in lumbar spine imaging which often does not extend far enough laterally to include the sacroiliac complex. Secondly pelvic tumours are hard to identify because of the presence of overlying intestinal gas (Bickels et al 1999). It is important that clinicians are not overly reliant on radiographic results in isolation as they can be misleading.

Grieve (1981) suggests the following indicators for the possibility of the presence of neoplasm.

Possible symptoms:

TABLE 1.4 TIMESCALE OF CANCER TYPE AND MEDICAL INTERVENTION (GRIEVE 1994)

Disease	*Time to first GP consultation*
Osteosarcoma	6/52
Ewing's sarcoma	16/52
Chondrosarcoma	21/52
Disease	*Time to diagnosis*
Pelvic tumours	61/52

- mild, severe or catastrophic pain
- pain severe enough to be uninfluenced by the usual analgesics, and requiring morphine for more than 48 hours
- weakness of legs
- unsteadiness of gait
- backache with pronounced loss of hip flexor power
- shock, vomiting and loss of spinal function following a trivial trauma (may be pathological fracture)

Possible signs:

- deformity of the spine
- 'globally' rigid cervical spine
- painful and restricted movement of the back
- swelling of soft parts of the back
- paraplegia
- the combination of shoulder girdle pain with neurological signs in the distribution of C8–T1 and Horner's syndrome.

Pyogenic infections

These are pus-forming in nature and are significantly different from TB, both in causation and clinical presentation. Patients with pyogenic infections may remain relatively healthy with no raised temperature or associated muscle spasm. The majority of infections are of insidious onset and commonly there is a prolonged period of time between onset and diagnosis. Early diagnosis is reliant on tacit knowledge of these conditions. The spinal regions affected by osteomyelitis are reported as; lumbar 50% of cases, followed by thoracic and then cervical with less than 10% of cases (Wainwright 2001).

Pyogenic infections have been linked to urinary tract infection, drug addiction, diabetes and after cardiac or urinary catheterization. It is worth noting that drug addiction is present on the CSAG (1994) Red Flag list. There are three groups of pyogenic infections, which vary in their anatomical site of presentation:

- vertebral body
- disc
- epidural space.

Those affecting the vertebral body constitute 1% of osteomyelitis cases. Although less common, infections of the disc can in 40% of cases result in paraparesis or paraplegia. This percentage increases to 75–100% in cases of infection of the epidural space, often presenting in the form of an epidural abscess (Leong & Luk 1996).

The symptoms may be acute or chronic but the predominant symptom is pain which may refer to the abdomen or the legs. The most common causative organism is *Staphylococcus* (50%). The remaining 50% is made up of:

- *Streptococcus*
- *Proteus* and *Escherichia coli*
- *Pseudomonas*
- *Klebsiella*
- *Salmonella typhi*
- *Streptococcus pneumoniae*
- *Brucella* (Leong & Luk 1996).

A survey in Denmark found an incidence rate of just 5 cases of acute vertebral osteomyelitis per million of population per year (Krogsgard et al 1998).

Brucellosis

Brucellosis is an infection which affects the lumbar spine more than any other part of the body (Leong & Luk 1996). Cyriax (1982) refers to brucellosis in the United Kingdom as a condition primarily affecting farmers and veterinary surgeons from Wales or the Midlands. He goes on to describe the outstanding symptoms as being fatigue, breathlessness and sweating after minor exertion, headache and pain in the back. Leong & Luk (1996) suggest that it can also affect those dealing with livestock and their preparation. It is caused by the *Brucella* bacteria and is commonly transmitted through unpasteurized milk or dairy products.

Grieve (1994) lists brucellosis as having a variety of names including undulant fever, abortus fever and Malta fever. He reports that it occurs uncommonly in agricultural communities, in mild and obscure forms. Grieve warns that a farm worker, for example, may present with migraine and vague muscle pains, and clinicians in country districts should be aware of the possibility. Data for the European Union show that the incidence decreased by 56% between 1996 and 2000, falling to 0.63 per 100 000. Brucellosis is most common in the following European countries (European Commission 2004):

- Greece
- Portugal
- Spain
- Italy.

Clinicians in rural areas need to be aware of the possibility of this presentation; similarly physiotherapists in urban environments may need to be aware of patients who have travelled to the Mediterranean or who work in abattoirs.

Tuberculosis (TB)

Tuberculosis (TB) like cancer has afflicted humankind for centuries and is commonly a disease associated with poverty and poor living conditions. Human remains dating from the Neolithic age (4500 BC) show evidence of TB type damage to the spine. TB bone lesions have been identified in Egyptian remains, and wall paintings of the time illustrate marked spinal deformity consistent with that found in TB spine. Contemporary medical reports suggest that death associated with TB spine was a common outcome (McGrew 1985).

An historical perspective is important for an understanding of the role of poverty alleviation in causing changing patterns of death and disease; lung TB provides an excellent example. In England and Wales, figures from 1850 onwards show that there was a steady decrease in the mortality of lung tuberculosis (Fig. 1.1), long before the discovery of *Mycobacterium tuberculosis* by Robert Koch around 1880. Anti-tuberculosis drugs

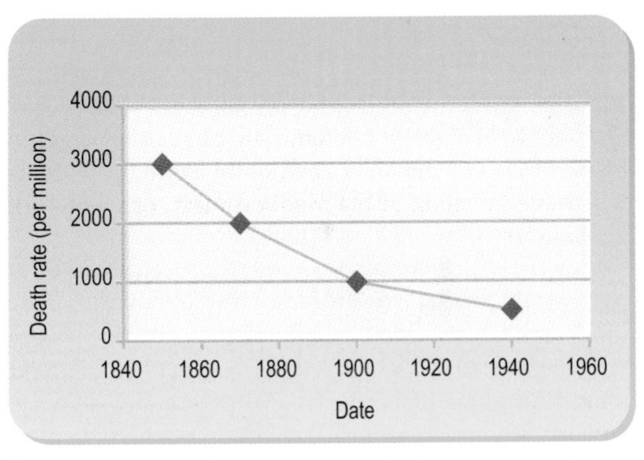

Figure 1.1 The declining death rate for TB of the lung, in England and Wales, before the introduction of vaccination. (Based on data in Bergstrom 1994.)

did not become widely used until the 1940s and the BCG vaccination came into public use later still. It is difficult to know exactly which factors were responsible for this decline. However, better housing, improved sanitation, declining illiteracy, better food, and generally improved standards of living are thought to have contributed (Bergstrom 1994).

Although poverty and poor living conditions are less common in developed industrial countries today, it is unfortunate that these conditions still exist in many parts of the world and still cause the spread of TB (Leong & Luk 1996). It was not until 50 years ago that the first medicines able to cure TB were developed. After a brief period of optimism the AIDS pandemic and the emergence of drug-resistant strains of the bacteria have resulted in TB re-emerging as a major threat to public health worldwide (WHO 2004b).

TB is a major health problem globally; overall 30% of the world's population is currently infected and someone in the world is newly infected with the bacterium every second (WHO 2004b). TB is described as a chronic, insidious and recurrent infection caused most commonly by *Mycobacterium tuberculosis* (Khoo et al 2003). Only people who are sick with pulmonary TB are infectious (WHO 2004b). Following treatment TB can remain dormant for as long as 30–40 years before recurrence (Leong & Luk 1996). TB infections of the spine are usually 'seeded' from the lungs (Khoo et al 2003). Interestingly, the most common spinal site of infection is the thoracolumbar junction (Wiesel et al 1996). Cyriax (1982) refers to this site as 'no man's land' and CSAG (1994) lists this area as a Red Flag.

In adults there are four primary patterns of spinal infection:

- paradiscal lesions
- anterior granuloma
- central lesions
- appendiceal type lesions.

Of these, paradiscal lesions are most common, representing approximately 50% of all cases (Khoo et al 2003).

Typical features of TB are backache with gibbus, an extreme kyphosis often with a marked angular deformity. Additional features may include abscess in the groin, trochanteric region or buttock (Leong & Luk 1996).

During the first half of the 20th century, TB started to decline due to the development of antibiotics. However, the combination of the development of antibiotic-resistant strains of the bacterium and the spread of HIV/AIDS has reversed this trend and prompted an increase in TB. A recent prospective survey conducted at the University Teaching Hospital, Zambia demonstrated an unusual pattern of admissions for spinal cord lesions. There were twice as many non-traumatic spinal cord lesions as there were traumatic lesions. TB spine was the most common reason for admission in the non-traumatic group, with 37 cases during a 5-month period (Mweemba 2005).

HIV/AIDS

HIV/AIDS are identified as Red Flags on the CSAG (1994) guidelines. The human immunodeficiency virus targets CD4+ T cells, a type of white blood cell, which is one of the key cells involved in fighting infection. The body's ability to fight disease decreases as the number of CD4+ T cells decreases. A healthy immune system has 800–1200 CD4+ T cells per cubic millimetre of blood; once this is reduced to 200 the patient is considered to have AIDS. As the immune system deteriorates it loses its capacity to fight disease and patients become increasingly susceptible to opportunistic illnesses (US Department of Health and Human Services 2004).

Regionally there are marked variations in the prevalence and incidence of HIV/AIDS. In the European Union there was a decrease in the annual incidence of 66% from 1994 to 2001; the cumulative total of AIDS cases for the EU in 2001 was 232 407 (European Commission 2004). In the United States AIDS-related deaths fell by 14% from 1998 to 2002, from 19 005 to 16 371 (US Department of Health and Human Services 2004). This is in stark contrast to the devastating AIDS pandemic in sub-Saharan Africa where approximately 25 million people are living with HIV/AIDS (US Department of Health and Human Services 2004). In Zambia alone it is estimated that 1 in 5 of the population is infected with the HIV virus and 200 people die of AIDS daily (Phiri 2004).

The diagnosis of AIDS, in an HIV-positive patient, requires the presence of at least one of the following opportunistic illnesses (European Commission 2004, Terence Higgins Trust 2004):

- pneumonia (present in 21–22% of cases)
- oesophageal candidiasis (present in 13–14.9% of cases)
- TB (present in 21.6% of cases)
- Kaposi's sarcoma (present in 5.5% of cases)
- toxoplasmosis.

Common symptoms occurring in people with AIDS (US Department of Health and Human Services 2004)

- Coughing and shortness of breath
- Lack of coordination
- Difficult or painful swallowing
- Mental symptoms such as confusion
- Severe and persistent diarrhoea
- Fever
- Vision loss
- Nausea and vomiting
- Weight loss
- Extreme fatigue
- Severe headaches

The relationship between HIV and TB is a synergistic one, in which their combined effect is worse than their separate effects added together (Tarantola & Mann 1994). For example, up to 60% of HIV-positive TB patients will have skeletal involvement compared to the usual 1% or 2% in HIV-negative patients (Khoo et al 2003).

CONCLUSION/SUMMARY

Despite the serious subject of this book it is vitally important for physiotherapists to retain a sense of perspective when examining and treating spinal patients. Physiotherapists need to recognize that serious pathology forms only a tiny proportion of the total caseload (Fig. 1.2).

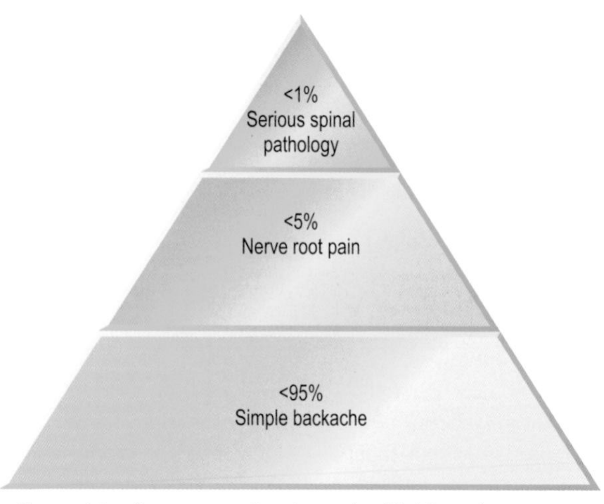

Figure 1.2 Percentage of patients classified into the diagnostic triage groups.

In addition, physiotherapists must not be alarmist as many patients present with some Red Flags in the presence of completely benign conditions. Over-medicalization and investigation of benign pathology can cause the patient a great deal of distress. The physiotherapist has a professional duty of care not to cause needless anxiety and concern for patients and their families.

The purpose of this book is to help differentiate between the small number of serious pathologies and the vast majority of benign conditions. The book will go on to discuss the sensitivity and specificity of Red Flags

Serious pathology correctly diagnosed
Serious pathology misdiagnosed as benign
Benign pathology misdiagnosed as serious
Benign pathology correctly diagnosed

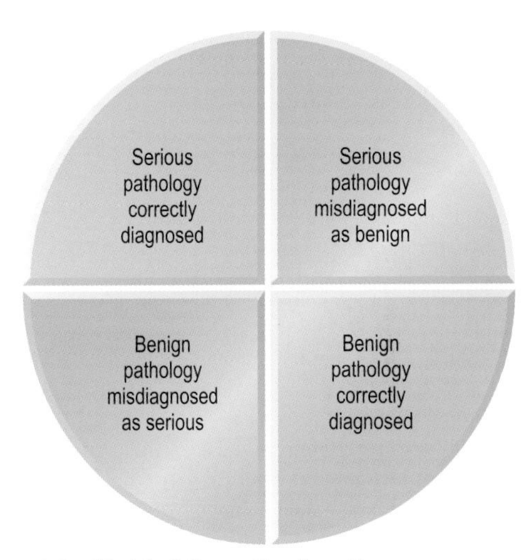

Figure 1.3 Model of diagnostic alternatives.

in the assessment of spinal conditions. This is graphically illustrated in Figure 1.3. Appropriate clinical reasoning will hopefully lead clinicians to an accurate diagnosis represented by the top left or bottom right quadrants in the figure.

References

Australian Department of Health and Ageing 2004 Cancer Data and Trends. Online. Available: http://www.health.gov.au 3 Aug 2004

Barclay J 1994 In good hands; The history of the Chartered Society of Physiotherapy 1894–1994. Butterworth Heinemann, Oxford

Bergstrom S 1994 The pathology of poverty. In: Lankinen et al K S (eds) Health and disease in developing countries. Macmillan Press, London, p 3–12

Bickels J, Kahanovitz N, Rubert C K et al 1999 Extraspinal bone and soft-tissue tumours as a cause of sciatica. Spine 24(15):1611–1616

Bigos S. 1994, Acute low back pain in adults: Clinical practice guideline, US Department of Health and Human Services, Rockville, MD. AHCPR 95-0643

Boissonnault W G 1995 Examination in physical therapy practice: screening for medical disease, 2nd edn. Churchill Livingstone, New York

Brewerton D A 2001 The doctor's role in diagnosis and prescribing vertebral manipulation. In: Maitland G et al (eds) Maitland's vertebral manipulation, 6th edn. Butterworth Heinemann, Oxford, p 16–20

CSAG 1994 Report of a Clinical Standards Advisory Group on Back Pain. HMSO, London

CSP 2004 Extended scope practitioners. Online. Available: http://www.csp.org.uk

Cyriax J 1982 Textbook of orthopaedic medicine, 8th edn. Baillière Tindall, Eastbourne

Department of Health 2000a Referral guidelines for suspected cancer. London

Department of Health 2000b The NHS plan. HMSO, London

European Commission 2004 Health statistics. Key data on health 2002 (data 1970–2001). European Commission

European Union 2004 European guidelines for prevention in low back pain. Online. Available: http://www.backpaineurope.org 28 Jan 2005

Gifford L 2000 The nerve root. CNS Press, Falmouth

Goodman C C, Fuller K S, Boissonnault W G 1998 Pathology implications for physical therapists, 2nd edn. Saunders, Philadelphia

Greenhalgh S, Selfe J 2004 Margaret: a tragic case of spinal Red Flags and Red Herrings. Physiotherapy 90(2):73–76 (also available at http://evolve.elsevier.com/Greenhalgh/redflags/)

Grieve G P 1981 Common vertebral joint problems. Churchill Livingstone, Edinburgh

Grieve G P 1994 'The masqueraders. In: Boyling J D, Palastanga N (eds) Grieve's modern manual therapy: the vertebral column, 2nd edn. Churchill Livingstone, Edinburgh, p 841–856

Kendall N A S, Linton S J, Main C 1997 Guide to assessing psychosocial yellow flags in acute low back pain: Risk factors for long term disability and work loss. Accident Rehabilitation and Compensation Insurance Corporation of New Zealand and the National Health Committee, Wellington

Khoo L T, Mikawa K, Fessler R G 2003 A surgical revisitation of Pott distemper of the spine. Spine Journal 3:130–145

Krogsgard M R, Wagn P, Bergtsson J 1998 Epidemiology of acute vertebral osteomyelitis in Denmark. Acta Orthopaedica Scandinavica 69:513–517

Leong J C Y, Luk K D K 1996 Spinal Infections. In: Wiesel S W et al (eds) The lumbar spine, International Society for the Study of the Lumbar Spine, 2nd edn. Saunders, Philadelphia, p 874–915

McGrew R E 1985 Encyclopedia of medical history. Macmillan Press, London

McKenzie R A 1990 The cervical and thoracic spine. Mechanical diagnosis and therapy. Spinal Publications, Waikanae

McKenzie R A, May S 2003 The lumbar spine. Mechanical diagnosis and therapy, Vol 1. Spinal Publications, Waikanae

Mennell J 1949 The science and art of joint manipulation: the extremities, 2nd edn. J & A Churchill, London

Mennell J 1952 The science and art of manipulation: the spinal column. J & A Churchill, London

Mweemba C 2005 Spinal cord injuries in Zambia BSc Dissertation Department of Physiotherapy University of Zambia

Mweemba C, Mwango M, Rochester P, Selfe J 2005 Spinal cord injuries in Zambia. International Journal of Therapy and Rehabilitation, in press

New Zealand Ministry of Health 2004 New Zealand Acute Low Back Pain Guidelines. Online. Available: http://www.nzgg.org.nz 4 Apr 2005

Ombregt L, Bisschop P, ter Veer H J 2003 A system of orthopaedic medicine, 2nd edn. Churchill Livingstone, London

Pfalzer L A 1995 Oncology: Examination, diagnosis and treatment. Medical and surgical considerations. In: Myers R S (ed) Saunders manual of physical therapy practice. Saunders, Philadelphia, p 65

Phiri M 2004 HIV/AIDS in Zambia WCPT Africa. 5th Regional Conference, Lusaka, Zambia

Ratliff J K, Cooper P R 2004 Metastatic spine tumours. Southern Medical Journal 97(3):246–253

Roberts P 1994 Theoretical models of physiotherapy. Physiotherapy 80(6):361–366

Royal College of General Practitioners 2001 Clinical guidelines for the management of acute low back pain. Online. Available: http://www.rcgp.org.uk/clinspec/guidelines/backpain/index.asp

Spitzer W O 1987 Quebec Task Force report. Spine 12(Suppl 1):S1–S59

Tarantola T, Mann J 1994 The AIDS pandemic. In: Lankinen K S et al (eds) Health and disease in developing countries. Macmillan Press, London, p 185–194

Terence Higgins Trust 2004 Toxoplasmosis information for people with HIV and AIDS. London

Thackray Museum 2004 Victorian Collection. Online. Available: www.thackraymuseum.org 22 Oct 2004

US Department of Health and Human Services 2004 How HIV causes AIDS. Online. Available: http://www.niaid.nih.gov/factsheets 3 Aug 2004

Waddell G 2004 The back pain revolution, 2nd edn. Churchill Livingstone, Edinburgh

Wainwright A 2001 Spinal infection. In: Bartley R, Coffey P (eds) Management of low back pain in primary care. Butterworth Heinemann, Oxford, p 99

WHO 2004a Cancer. Online. Available: http:www.who.int/cancer 22 Apr 2004

WHO 2004b Tuberculosis infection and transmission. Online. Available: http://www.who.int/mediacentre/factsheets/fs104/en/ 104 22 Apr 2004

Wiesel S W, Weinstein J N, Herkowitz H et al 1996 The lumbar spine, International Society for the Study of the Lumbar Spine, 2nd edn. Saunders, Philadelphia

Chapter 2

Clinical Reasoning

CHAPTER CONTENTS

One of the many clinical challenges facing physiotherapists is the issue of diagnosis of spinal pain. There are numerous causes of spinal pain, and a multitude of individual anatomical structures either individually or in combination can contribute to the clinical symptom of spinal pain.

Potential causes of spinal pain

- Structural abnormalities
- Inflammatory processes
- Degenerative processes
- Infective processes
- Neoplastic processes
- Metabolic processes
- Visceral referral
- Idiopathic

However, in the quest for a diagnosis it is vitally important to remember that back pain is actually just a symptom, not a disease, and that a diagnosis of specific pathology is only achievable in about 15% of cases of spinal pain (Waddell 2004).

The International Association for the Study of Pain (IASP) defines pain as 'an unpleasant sensory and *emotional experience* associated with actual or potential tissue damage or described in terms of such damage' (Merskey & Bogduk 1994, emphasis ours).

Using this IASP definition of pain helps us to understand that pain is much more than a 'simple' nociceptive output from injured tissue but is in fact a very complex sensory and emotional experience. Gifford & Butler (1997) suggest that clinicians should consider pain as three interacting dimensions:

- sensory–discriminative: awareness of intensity, location, quality and pain behaviour
- cognitive–evaluative: thoughts about the problem influenced by experiences and previous knowledge
- motivational–affective: the emotional response (often negative) that motivates or governs response to pain, e.g. fear, anxiety or anger.

By adopting a clinical approach that incorporates both physical and psychosocial factors, physiotherapists align themselves with the holistic philosophy of patient care encouraged by the WHO International Classification of Functioning, Disability and Health (WHO 2001).

PAIN, BEHAVIOUR AND PSYCHOSOCIAL FLAGS

We have so far exclusively discussed physical problems. However, it is important to remember the very complex emotional and psychological reactions that can accompany even simple mechanical spinal pain. Current research evidence suggests strong links between psychological variables and spinal pain (Linton 2000, Sterling 2004). Current evidence suggests that some psychological variables may also have a genetic link (MacGregor et al 2004). A flag system highlighting risk factors has been developed to alert the clinician that there may be a risk of poor outcome due to low back pain for reasons other than biomedical ones. Chapter 1 traces the development of the Red Flag system of biomedical indicators of serious pathology. The following flag system highlights psychosocial indicators (C Main, personal communication, 2005, Main & Williams 2002, Schultz & Gatchel 2005):

- Yellow Flags – emotional and behavioural factors
- Blue Flags – social and economic factors
- Black Flags – occupational factors
- Orange Flags – psychiatric factors.

Grieve (1981) points out that continuous and harrowing distress can be the dominant feature of pain from malignancy; an emotionally disturbed patient with psychogenic pain may give the same impression. However, in the latter case the patient tends to describe suffering rather than symptoms. The extravagance of the description of painful suffering may invite the suspicion that while the patient may be in pain, the kind of help they need is not that indicated for malignant disease. Emotional and psychological issues associated with spinal pain are addressed in detail by Gordon Waddell in his book *The Back Pain Revolution* (Waddell 2004) and in the New Zealand 'Guide to assessing psychosocial Yellow Flags in acute low back pain' (New Zealand Ministry of Health 2002).

Both publications highlight the complexity of these emotional and psychological reactions and propose that clinicians should use a biopsychosocial model of illness as a framework when interpreting the complex picture of the patient's physical and emotional presentation. Roberts (2000) argues that Red and Yellow Flags are not mutually exclusive; the complexity of cases in which both are present poses a significant challenge. It must be considered that those with serious pathology can develop increased psychosocial stresses as the condition progresses, especially in view of the delay in detection (for example, see 'Cancer' section in Ch. 1). Three-dimensional thinking (see Fig. 2.2) is hugely important in these cases, to help differentiate between apparently serious or genuinely serious presentations (Fig. 2.1).

In addition, Waddell (2004) also identifies a group of patients with low back pain who demonstrate very overt pain behaviour. These patients display an exaggerated pain behaviour which can manifest in a number of ways. One of the problems facing clinicians is that these overt pain behaviours can often be the same as those displayed by patients with serious pathology.

The following extract helps to illustrate this:

> *He moved to a chair in reception and sat down and soon began to half lie on to the next chair. Within two minutes he stood up and leaned against a cupboard.* (Greenhalgh & Selfe 2003)

Waddell (2004) cites the University of Alabama (UAB) pain behaviour scale as a useful tool in helping clinicians determine the degree of pain behaviour (Richards et al 1982). The scale consists of ten items; with reference to the clinical example above it is interesting to consider two of the ten items:

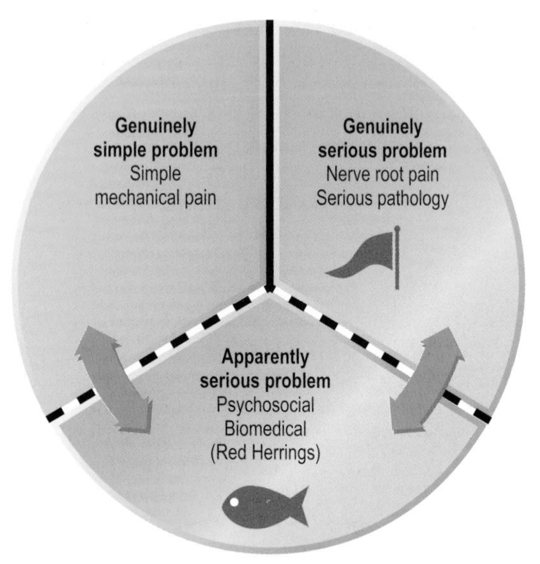

Figure 2.1 Model differentiating between genuinely simple, apparently serious and genuinely serious problems.

- item eight: 'Use of physical supports (corset, stick, crutches, lean on furniture, transcutaneous electrical nerve stimulation (TENS) – none; occasional; dependent; constant use)'
- item nine: 'Stationary movement (sit or stand still; occasional shift of position; constant movement or shifts of position)'.

The patient described would score highly on these two items of the UAB scale. However, the patient did not have an exaggerated reaction to his pain; he was diagnosed with a malignant myeloma of T12 and subsequently underwent a vertebrectomy (Greenhalgh & Selfe 2003). With respect to this difficult issue Waddell (2004) urges caution and states that clinicians should:

> *Always carry out diagnostic triage first. Exclude serious spinal pathology or a widespread neurological disorder before even thinking about illness behaviour.*

This is a view that we would strongly endorse.

Not many figures are available on the incidence of overt pain behaviour in the back pain population. Waddell et al (1980) reported an incidence rate of 10% among patients referred to an orthopaedic clinic from general practitioners in the UK. Also in the UK, Selfe (1995) reported that 8% of patients from a sample of 300 low back pain patients referred to physiotherapy via general practitioners, orthopaedic consultants and rheumatology consultants demonstrated sufficiently overt pain behaviour to require referral to a specialist multidisciplinary pain management programme. It must be remembered that a patient chronically disabled for many decades with low back pain is not immune from serious pathology.

The importance of the biopsychosocial approach to low back pain was highlighted in the CSAG guidelines (CSAG 1994). Biopsychosocial issues have been highlighted as contributory factors in spinal pain becoming chronic, increasing the risk of long-term disability and social exclusion (CSAG 1994). Traditionally physiotherapists have not routinely measured psychosocial risk, in a formal way. The Linton and Halden Initial Back Pain Questionnaire (L&H questionnaire or acute low back pain screening questionnaire) was specifically developed to measure psychosocial risk factors in patients with low back pain (Waddell 2004). The L&H questionnaire is now widely used by physiotherapists. Hurley et al (2001) report that the final total score on the L&H questionnaire correlated with pain and disability at 1-year follow-up. However, high L&H scores can also be obtained purely by severe pain unrelated to significant psychosocial issues (Greenhalgh et al 2005). The L&H questionnaire should therefore be used as one of a number of aids in clinical decision-making.

In addition to formal questionnaires, Waddell (2004) also suggests a mnemonic for clinicians, to guide them through topics to explore during the subjective history-taking of biopsychosocial issues: A, B, C, D, E, F, W.

- A – Attitudes and beliefs about pain
- B – Behaviours
- C – Compensation issues
- D – Diagnosis and treatment issues
- E – Emotions
- F – Family
- W – Work.

A more detailed discussion of these important psychosocial issues is beyond the scope of a pocket guide to Red Flags; interested readers are referred to the work of Linton (2000), Main & Williams (2002) and Waddell (2004).

As described in the previous chapter, a number of reports have produced simplified diagnostic schemes in an attempt to aid clinicians. The Quebec Task Force produced a list of 11 diagnostic categories (Spitzer 1987). CSAG (1994) described five diagnostic categories for spinal disorders, which was further condensed into the diagnostic triage:

- simple backache (95% of cases)
- nerve root pain (<5% of cases)
- possible serious spinal pathology (<1% of cases).

These diagnostic categories are intended to help clinicians and to simplify diagnosis, and indeed the diagnostic triage appears very successful in this regard as it provides a clear framework for clinical decision-making. However, even using a simple tool such as the diagnostic triage can be challenging; this is illustrated in Figure 2.1.

There should be little difficulty distinguishing between genuinely simple problems and those that are genuinely serious; this is denoted by the solid line. However, the dashed lines show where diagnostic difficulty may occur around the apparently serious problems which often present with very complex clinical pictures.

CLINICAL REASONING

Clinical reasoning refers to the thought processes used in patient diagnosis and management and is universally applied by clinicians. Jones & Rivett (2004) suggest that while conceptually very simple, clinical reasoning in practice is actually very difficult and fraught with errors. They state that 'therapists must be able to think along multiple lines and often think on different levels at the same time'. This is a point we would strongly agree with. To illustrate the complexity of clinical reasoning we use the term three-dimensional thinking (3D thinking; Fig. 2.2). 3D thinking is a very dynamic and rapidly occurring process. 3D thinking should permit a unique therapist response (output) in relation to each individual and unique patient scenario (input).

Figure 2.2 also shows how equal weight is placed on the patient (input) and the physiotherapist (output). This illustrates that for clinical reasoning to be successful the patient and therapist should form an active and balanced partnership in trying to come to an understanding of the patient's condition. It is also important to note that the vertical line in the centre of Figure 2.2 has an arrowhead at both ends. This illustrates that during patient consultations physiotherapists draw on their previous experience and knowledge and that simultaneously each patient consultation adds to the physiotherapist's knowledge and experience.

Central to clinical reasoning is the concept of clinicians reflecting or thinking about their own thought processes when engaged in patient contact; this is

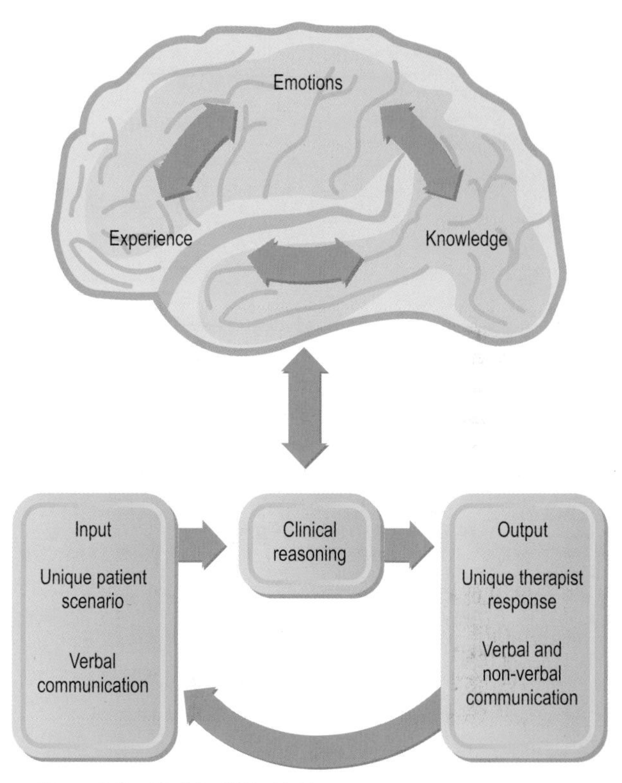

Figure 2.2 Model of 3D thinking.

referred to as metacognition. Rather than being a passive or theoretical activity, metacognition should be an ongoing dynamic and practical activity underpinning all clinical reasoning. There are a number of elements to metacognition, including:

- metacognitive knowledge: thinking about knowledge
- metacognitive skill: thinking about current action (Hacker 1998).

To underline the universality and importance of clinical reasoning in the clinical environment Schell (1998) suggests that: 'It is not a question of whether you are doing it, only a question of how well'.

Clearly clinical reasoning is a very important process in the day-to-day practice of a wide variety of professions; from a physiotherapy perspective Jones (1995) lists three reasons why it is so important:

- It provides a safeguard against the risk of popular theory and practice being accepted without question.
- Without clinical reasoning clinical practice becomes merely a technical operation.
- It is important in avoiding misdirection in beliefs and helps to manage the rapidly expanding body of clinical and biomedical knowledge.

Schell (1998) describes four categories of clinical reasoning:

- scientific
- narrative

- pragmatic
- ethical.

According to Edwards et al (2004), clinical reasoning has mainly developed from a quantitative scientific perspective set within a positivistic paradigm and has primarily been concerned with diagnosis (diagnostic reasoning). Within the diagnostic reasoning model, two distinct processes of clinical reasoning have been identified:

- hypothetico-deductive reasoning, used primarily by more inexperienced practitioners or by experts when faced with unfamiliar or complex presentations
- pattern recognition, which is faster and more efficient and is used by experienced and expert practitioners.

Jones & Rivett (2004) explain that these processes involve collecting and analysing information and hypothesis generation about the cause or nature of the patient's condition. This begins with the therapist's observation and interpretation of initial cues from the patient when they first meet, even before any verbal communication takes place. The following extract from Greenhalgh & Selfe (2003) helps to illustrate this point:

> *John was a 64-year-old man leaning heavily on the reception desk and obviously in a great deal of discomfort when first seen, but was trying hard to smile. He appeared unwell with a sallow complexion, slightly dishevelled appearance and poorly fitting clothes. He moved to a chair in reception and sat down and soon*

began to half lie on to the next chair. Within two minutes he stood up and leaned against a cupboard.

There is a wealth of non-verbal information that can be gained from this description and it shows how the therapist should be able to develop an initial concept of the problem that includes preliminary working hypotheses for considering during the examination. In this example it is clear that the patient is displaying marked illness behaviour; two alternative hypotheses that could explain this behaviour can be formulated:

- The patient has an abnormal and exaggerated reaction to a minor problem.
- The patient has a normal reaction to a very severe and painful problem.

In the hypothetico-deductive reasoning model these hypotheses are tested through further data collection to determine optimal treatment and management strategies based on these data.

Hypothesis categories (Jones & Rivett 2004)

- Activity capability or restriction
- Patients' perspectives on their experience
- Pathobiological mechanisms
- Physical impairments
- Contributing factors
- Precautions and contraindications
- Management and treatment
- Prognosis

Although we have used a fairly simple example above, patients sometimes present with very complex problems where multiple competing hypotheses can be generated. This is particularly true in cases of serious spinal pathology. In these cases it is worth remembering and adopting the principle of parsimony (sometimes referred to as Ockham's razor) first attributed to the 14th century logician and Franciscan friar, William of Ockham:

> *Of two competing theories or explanations, all other things being equal, the simpler one is to be preferred.* (Chalmers 2003)

This is commonly expressed as 'If you hear the sound of hooves outside you should assume it is a horse not a zebra' (Fig. 2.3).

The physician Sir Arthur Conan Doyle, creator of Sherlock Holmes, was an advocate of the principle of parsimony. He states '. . . when you have eliminated the impossible, whatever remains, however improbable, must be the truth'. He also suggests that logic must prevail (Dillin & Watkins 1992); therefore when applying the principle of parsimony to serious spinal pathology it is vitally important for physiotherapists to remember that serious pathology accounts for no more than 1% of all back pain (CSAG 1994).

Using the horse/zebra illustration it is also possible to consider how one would confirm whether a horse or a zebra is outside, i.e. one would need to look out of the window to gather more information. Jones (1992) argues that successful clinical reasoning does precisely this. It

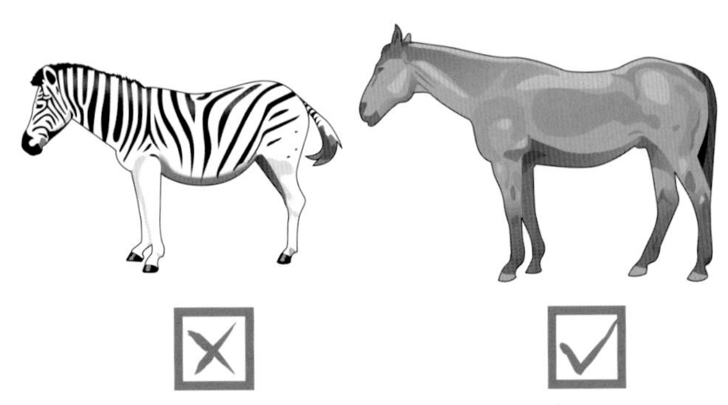

Figure 2.3 'If you hear the sound of hooves outside you should assume it is a horse not a zebra.'

is a process of ongoing data collection, and does not stop on completion of the assessment; continuous reassessment is essential and contributes to the therapist's evolving concept of the patient's problem.

In a paper that demonstrates a clear link between diagnostic reasoning and its positivistic origins, Round (2000) suggests that clinicians should utilize Bayes' theorem as an aid to diagnosis. Thomas Bayes was an 18th century mathematician, and his theorem concerns conditional probabilities. According to Chalmers (2003) these are:

Probabilities for propositions that depend on (and hence are conditional on) the evidence bearing on those propositions.

Put another way, the probability ascribed to an event depends on prior knowledge of the event and if any new evidence pertaining to the circumstances of the event comes to light the probability (related to the event) changes in response to the new evidence.

In the horse/zebra example used above, the conditional probabilities partly depend on where you live; generally in the North West of England zebras would have a very low probability; however, the conditional probability can change. The city of Chester provides an example:

- living next door to Chester Zoo (zebra possible)
- living next door to Chester Race Course (horse very likely).

From a clinical perspective this could very simply be expressed as keeping an open mind about the patient's condition and being prepared to modify ideas in response to any new information that comes to light. This reinforces the earlier point made by Jones & Rivett (2004) that successful clinical reasoning involves a continuous process of reassessment and an evolving concept of the patient's problem.

In practical terms the way conditional probabilities can influence clinical decision-making is illustrated by the following examples. The International Myeloma Foundation suggests that there is a rare tendency for myeloma to have a genetic link (3–5% of cases). However, it is also likely that a combination of several environmental and predisposing factors can culminate in the development of myeloma.

Predisposing factors for myeloma (International Myeloma Foundation 2002)

- African descent
- Exposure to chemicals (dioxins and solvents)
- Exposure to radiation
- Viral infection (HIV, hepatitis, herpes and cytomegalovirus)
- Age 50–70

Therefore the conditional probability is affected by the presence, absence or combination of these factors. Interestingly, Durie (2004) reports a trend toward an increased incidence of myeloma below the age of 55 years. He suggests this may be due to changing environmental factors over the last 30–40 years.

Similarly, environmental factors and genetically linked predisposing factors can have an effect on breast cancer. A recent study revealed that among women who smoked for 20 years or longer there was a 60% increase in the incidence of breast cancer. Among those who smoked 20 cigarettes a day or more for 40 years, the risk rose to 83% (Terry et al 2002).

Returning to Bayes' theorem, Round (2000) proposes a more formal use of the theorem in relation to diagnostic reasoning. She advocates that clinicians could use the theorem as the basis on which to calculate the likelihood ratios of a particular medical condition. In order to calculate likelihood ratios it is necessary to know two things about an item of clinical information; these are:

- the specificity, the chance of having a negative result when the disease is absent
- the sensitivity, the chance of having a positive result when the disease is present.

One of the challenges facing physiotherapists is that the specificity and sensitivity of many of the objective tests used in clinical practice have not been established. This issue has recently been highlighted in the UK and research into the physical diagnostic tests commonly used by physiotherapists has become a research funding priority (CSP 2002). This problem, however, is not just restricted to the UK. Interested readers are directed to McKenzie & May (2003a, 2003b) who, drawing from a wide international literature, provide a comprehensive review and discussion on this subject. In light of the problems associated with objective examination, it is interesting, and somewhat reassuring, to note that according to Deyo et al (1992) the objective examination is actually much less useful than the subjective examination in identifying serious pathology in the early stages. The patient's own story of their lived experience provides valuable and rich diagnostic data which should never be underestimated or ignored. It is not until the later stages of the disease that objective markers of progressing pathology become evident.

Deyo et al (1992) report that during history-taking a variety of subjective markers have been shown to have high specificity and sensitivity. For example, a previous medical history of cancer has a specificity of 0.98. Frymoyer (1997) agrees with this view and reports that any history of a known primary cancer, however remote, should be considered significant. Both these reports suggest that in patients with histories of previous cancer the conditional probability is very high and that there may be a recurrence at some stage. Clinicians need to be aware of this and remain vigilant. Therefore during the clinical decision-making process, screening questions for recurrent cancer should take place at the initial stages.

Wardle et al (2005) illustrate this point in the case of Christine, a 53-year-old patient who had a previous history of acute myeloid leukaemia who presented with what initially appeared to be a frozen shoulder 20 years later. This patient was ultimately diagnosed with a brachial plexus granulocytic sarcoma. In a study of almost 2000 patients suffering from back pain, no cancer was identified in any patient below the age of 50 years without a previous history of cancer, unexplained weight loss or failed previous intervention (Deyo et al 1992).

KEY FACT: The sensitivity of these four combined markers, previous cancer, age, weight loss and failed conservative management, is 1.00 (a staggering 100%).

Many clinicians would tend to assume that the sensitivity of weight loss was high. However, Deyo et al (1992) state that the sensitivity is 0.15 and the specificity

0.94 for diagnostic accuracy of weight loss in the medical history. It is also important to remember that in some conditions, for example myeloma, weight loss may not occur until later stages of the disease process (Durie 2004). Weight loss in the later stage of cancer is termed cachexia and is defined as a wasting syndrome in which fat and muscle tissue are lost; it is indicative of a state of malnutrition (Maltzman 2004), and is discussed further in Chapter 4.

Osteoporosis is another condition where conditional probability is dependent on knowledge of the combination of presenting factors. It is a common condition responsible for 40 000 clinically diagnosed fractures each year in the UK alone (Bolton Hospitals NHS Trust 1996). The estimated cost of care of osteoporotic fractures in postmenopausal women in the UK is estimated to be in the region of £1030 million (NICE 2005). Conditional probability in osteoporosis, for example, depends on:

- corticosteroid usage
- gender
- early menopause
- history of previous fracture
- family history of osteoporosis.

A patient taking systemic steroids who develops low back pain has a specificity of 0.99 when considering vertebral compression fractures (Dukes 2004). However, providing no fracture has occurred, once steroid treatment has been withdrawn the effects are reversible.

Another area of interest when considering conditional probabilities is spinal infection. Experience would suggest that the clinician often assumes that the presence of a fever (including night sweats) may indicate some sort of infection; conversely absence of a fever tends to reassure clinicians when considering spinal infection. Importantly, however, the sensitivity of fever in the case of tuberculous osteomyelitis is a mere 0.27. A fever therefore is suggestive, but not specific (Deyo et al 1992).

The model of diagnostic reasoning outlined above set within a positive paradigm has not been without criticism. Scott (2000) states that three types of error can occur:

1. faulty perception or elicitation of cues
2. incomplete factual knowledge
3. misapplication of known facts to a specific problem.

Downing & Hunter (2003) pick up on this first point when they point out that subjectivity is entwined with clinical reasoning. This is a problem associated with bias, which (Murphy 1997) defines as:

> *Any process at any stage of inference which tends to produce results or conclusions that differ systematically from the truth.*

Within clinical practice, bias can come from many sources and can occur at both a conscious and unconscious level. This can have serious consequences when considering patients' own self-diagnosis and misattribution; this is discussed more fully later in this chapter.

Both Schell (1998) and Edwards et al (2004) highlight that diagnostic reasoning set within a positive paradigm does not consider that many clinical tasks require an understanding of the person as well as the disease. They go on to point out that the world of the patient is both a biomedical and a lived experience. In order to address this issue narrative reasoning within a qualitative paradigm has developed. Narrative reasoning seeks to understand the unique lived experience of patients, a reasoning activity that could be termed the construction of meaning. It is essential that subjective questioning enables the clinician to understand the entire patient story.

Edwards et al (2004) develop this concept and propose a conceptual framework which considers the dialectical nature of reasoning. This acknowledges the legitimacy of different reasoning processes without attempting to establish the supremacy of one over the other. They go on to describe how in real life there is a dynamic interplay between different types of reasoning. They also argue, and are supported by Hack (2004), that this mode of thinking relates well to the biopsychosocial model of health (Waddell 2004) and the WHO International Classification of Functioning, Disability and Health (WHO 2001). A further extract of the case history presented earlier helps to illustrate this:

> *At home he needed the help of his 16-year old daughter to dress and undress.* (Greenhalgh & Selfe 2003)

Remembering that the patient being described is a 64-year-old male, this extract demonstrates how his spinal problem occurs in a unique social setting and how the spinal problem in turn actually impacts on and changes the social dynamic of his world. This role reversal is commonplace when functional activity is limited by a musculoskeletal disorder. It is vitally important that the physiotherapist recognizes that this information provides a valuable insight into the world of the patient's own experience and considers these issues when trying to understand the patient's problem and when formulating a suitable management plan. In this particular case, this information helped to contribute to a picture of a patient with a serious pathology.

Schell (1998) describes pragmatic reasoning and ethical reasoning. Pragmatic reasoning is 'the world in which therapy occurs'. This world has two components:

- Practice: this includes things such as treatment resources and organizational culture.
- Personal: this includes things such as clinical competence and demands outside of work.

These professional and personal issues can strongly influence clinical reasoning.

Scientific, narrative and pragmatic reasoning all attempt to answer questions about what is the patient's problem and what can be done to help that problem. Ethical reasoning asks the question 'What should be done?'.

Both pragmatic and ethical reasoning are important when managing patients with serious pathology, as the following extract illustrates.

> *These findings strongly suggested that John had serious pathology; his case was immediately discussed with the consultant adviser. John was admitted directly to an orthopaedic ward . . . Within a few hours John had received a magnetic resonance image scan and blood tests, which implied plasmacytoma (myeloma).*
>
> (Greenhalgh & Selfe 2003)

In this case the process of pragmatic reasoning by the physiotherapist was relatively easy; the organizational culture strongly supported her, and she could speak immediately to an orthopaedic consultant who was then able to initiate the admission and subsequent investigation process. It also highlights the ethical reasoning dimension of 'what should be done?'. As the physiotherapist was highly suspicious that the patient had serious pathology, ethically it was imperative to seek a further opinion.

HEALTH BEHAVIOUR

Within musculoskeletal practice it is useful to consider why patients seek treatment. The simple answer is usually associated with pain that is negatively impacting on some aspect of the patient's function. However, the issue is rarely that simple and a whole academic discipline of health psychology has developed in order to answer some of the more complex issues surrounding health behaviour.

Conner & Norman (1995) provide a detailed critical review of some of the key concepts in health psychology and explore how these inform us about health-related behaviours. They state that social cognition is concerned with how individuals make sense of a variety of social situations. A number of social cognition models have been developed to explain health-related behaviours and subsequent responses to treatment. They provide a basis for understanding the determinants of behaviour and behaviour change.

The five main models of health behaviour (Conner & Norman 1995)

- Health belief model
- Health locus of control
- Protection motivation theory
- Theory of planned behaviour
- Self-efficacy model

It is beyond the scope of this pocket guide to provide a detailed analysis of these models. However; with reference to serious spinal pathology a brief discussion of the health belief model provides a useful insight into a patient's behaviour in response to illness. The central tenet of this model is that the threat of illness determines health behaviour. The health belief model is made up of six independent predictors of behaviour.

Health belief model (Conner & Norman 1995)

- Perceptions of illness threat (serious/benign)
- Evaluation of behaviours to counteract this threat (action/no action)
- Perceived susceptibility to the illness (vulnerability)
- Perceived severity of the consequences of such illness (prognosis)
- Cues to action either external (media) or internal (physical symptom)
- Health motivation (value placed on health)

Together these variables determine behaviour. Individuals are likely to follow a particular health action if they believe themselves to be susceptible to a particular condition, which they also consider to be serious, and if they believe that the benefits of the action taken to counteract the health threat outweigh the costs.

This is particularly important in cases of serious spinal pathology as outcome of treatment is often dependent on stage of condition, so that earlier diagnoses are very often associated with better outcomes (Canadian Strategy for Cancer Control 2002). Cancer that has metastasized is rarely curable (Jarvik & Deyo 2002). The difficulty here is that in the early stages it can be very difficult to identify the presence of serious pathology. Patients at this early stage will tend to have a low perception of illness threat and will also tend to have a low perceived severity of the consequences of their problem; as a result they are probably less likely to seek an early medical opinion. Although entirely understandable, the patient's behaviour at this stage may actually contribute to a poorer outcome later in the disease process.

There are also important gender issues involved in this issue, as a MORI poll in 1994 identified that male patients seek medical intervention much later than females (Banks 1997); this is regardless of income or ethnicity (Banks 2001).

One of the key factors involved in this complex picture revolves around the patient's own self-diagnosis of their condition. Leventhal & Crouch (1997) suggest that a patient's behaviour is determined by his or her own self-diagnosis. This self-diagnosis is determined by mapping the signs and symptoms of the health problem against five attributes, described by Leventhal et al (1997).

Self-diagnosis model (Leventhal et al 1997)

- Disease identity (diagnostic label)
- Timeline (acute versus chronic)
- Consequences (prognosis/likely outcome)
- Causes (reasons/blame)
- Controllability (is intervention necessary?)

The challenge for clinicians is to assess whether the patient's self-diagnosis is accurate. Wiesel et al (1996) report: 'Patients often relate their pain to a fall or some other mishap.' Wilson (2002) also highlights that inappropriate attribution by patients of insidious symptoms to a traumatic event is common and can be very misleading. In a previous paper we have used the term Red Herring to describe this and any other misleading aspects of the patient's history or presentation (Greenhalgh & Selfe 2004). The following extract is taken from a case we used to illustrate the point.

> *Margaret attributed symptoms to her road traffic accident and indeed the site of symptoms was consistent with mechanical injury, where Margaret was in the driver's seat and the driver's door was the point of impact of the motorcyclist.*

In Margaret's self-diagnosis scheme, the mechanical trauma of the road traffic accident was considered to be the cause of her symptoms (predominantly right rib pain); unfortunately this was a Red Herring. Margaret in fact had widespread metastatic disease secondary to primary breast cancer. The difficulty of Margaret's case lies in the fact that to a physiotherapist Margaret's own self-diagnosis seemed as if it was highly accurate. However, it is vital that all other available information is assessed, as that may cast a different light on the problem.

SUMMARY

In Chapter 1 we reviewed the development of a number of influential reports on back pain management;

contained within these have been a number of Red Flag lists. In this chapter we have reviewed clinical decision-making processes and in particular have discussed conditional probabilities. Although the Red Flag lists are very useful, one thing they do not provide clinicians with, which would be extremely useful, is a hierarchy of the importance of each Red Flag either singly or in groups. When considering the previous discussion on conditional probabilities we feel this is an important point for clinicians. To illustrate this point consider the following scenarios:

1. A 49-year-old woman involved in a road traffic accident presents with thoracic pain and no previous history of cancer.
2. A 63-year-old woman involved in a road traffic accident presents with thoracic pain and no previous history of cancer.
3. A 49-year-old woman involved in a road traffic accident presents with thoracic pain with a previous history of cancer.
4. A 63-year-old woman involved in a road traffic accident presents with thoracic pain with a previous history of cancer.

Scenarios 1 and 2 are very similar, both have the Red Flags of road traffic accident and thoracic pain; the only difference is the age of the patient. What is interesting is that the age of the patient in scenario 2 is now also a Red Flag. When the age changes to a Red Flag the conditional probability changes; however, most clinicians would probably not be unduly alarmed by this. Now consider the difference between scenarios 3 and 4. Here we have the same change in age of the patient but set against a background of previous history of cancer; here the effect of age has a more pronounced effect on clinical decision-making.

Now compare the differences between scenario 1 and 3 and then scenario 2 and 4. These pairs of scenarios are similar but note the effect of the addition of previous history of cancer. Each time previous history of cancer is present it appears to have a greater impact on clinical decision-making than age, even though they are both Red Flags in this instance. Clinicians need to take this factor into account during clinical decision-making.

The point we are making here is that clearly the conditional probabilities change across all four of the scenarios but what is unknown is by how much. Which individual Red Flags and which combinations are most important? Roberts (2000) identifies '. . . a surprisingly poor evidence base for danger signs'. Roberts (2000) provides a suggested hierarchy of danger signs which was proposed following a review of the literature and the experience of a multidisciplinary research team:

- probable danger signs; indicative of serious spinal pathology
- possible danger signs; evidence more controversial
- probably not danger signs; little or no evidence.

Hierarchy of danger signs (Roberts 2000)

Probable danger signs
- Extensor plantar response
- Neurological signs at multiple levels
- Saddle anaesthesia

Possible danger signs
- 'Constant' night pain
- Bilateral leg signs

Probably not danger signs
- Severe local back pain
- Loss of reflex at one level
- Unilateral sciatic symptoms below the knee

The following section presents our own weighted list of Red Flags which builds on and develops Roberts' earlier work. In the next three chapters we will expand on why it is important to identify these particular signs or symptoms, including a discussion on their sensitivity and specificity. We will also explore how they interact with each other and influence conditional probabilities; finally we will provide suggestions for strategies on how to deal with them if they are identified.

WEIGHTED RED FLAG LIST

Subjective examination: age, previous medical history and lifestyle questions (Ch. 3)

- Age
  <10 ⚑⚑⚑
  11–19 ⚑⚑
  20–50
  >51 ⚑⚑⚑
- Medical history (current or past) of ⚑⚑⚑
  Cancer
  TB
  HIV/AIDS or injection drug abuse
  Osteoporosis
- Smoking ⚑

Subjective examination: history of current episode questions (Ch. 4)

- Weight loss (3–6 months)
  Weight loss <5% body weight ⚑
  Weight loss 5–10% body weight ⚑⚑
  Weight loss >10% body weight ⚑⚑⚑
- Cauda equina syndrome ⚑⚑⚑
- Systemically unwell ⚑
- Trauma ⚑
- Vertebrobasilar insufficiency ⚑
- Bilateral pins and needles in hands and/or feet ⚑
- Previous failed treatment ⚑

Age >50 years + history of cancer + unexplained weight loss + failure to improve after 1 month of conservative therapy

Subjective examination: pain questions (Ch. 4)

- Constant progressive pain
- Thoracic pain
- Abdominal pain and changed bowel habits but with no change of medication
- Severe night pain
- Headache

Objective examination (Ch. 5)

- Physical appearance
- Inability to lie supine
- Bizarre neurological deficit
- Marked partial articular restriction of movement
- Loss of sphincter tone and altered S4 sensation
- Spasm
- Vertebral artery testing
- Upper cervical instability tests
- Positive extensor plantar response
- Disturbed gait

Red Herrings

- Misattribution by:
    - Patient

- Referring doctor or allied health professional
- Treating physiotherapist

- Inappropriate overt illness behaviour
- Other conditions which complicate the clinical scenario but which do not impact on the management of the patient
- Biomedical masqueraders

References

Banks I 1997 Men's health. The Black-Staff Press, Belfast

Banks I 2001 No man's land: men, illness and the NHS. BMJ 323:1058–1060

Bolton Hospitals NHS Trust 1996 Osteoporosis management: guidelines for the prevention, diagnosis and treatment of osteoporosis. Bolton

Canadian Strategy for Cancer Control 2002 Cancer diagnosis in Canada

Chalmers A F 2003 What is this thing called Science?, 3rd edn. Open University Press, Maidenhead

Conner M, Norman P 1995 Predicting health behaviour. Open University Press, Buckingham

CSAG 1994 Report of a Clinical Standards Advisory Group on Back Pain. HMSO, London

CSP 2002 Priorities for physiotherapy research in the UK: project report. CSP, London

Deyo R A, Rainville J, Kent D L 1992 What can the history and physical examination tell us about low back pain? JAMA 268(6):760–765

Dillin W H, Watkins R G 1992 Back pain in children and adolescents. In: Rothman R H, Simeone F A (eds) The spine, 3rd edn. Saunders, Philadelphia, p 231–259

Downing A M, Hunter D G 2003 Validating clinical reasoning: question of perspective, but whose perspective. Manual Therapy 8(2):117–119
Dukes M N G 2004 Myler's side effects of drugs, 14th edn. Elsevier, Amsterdam
Durie B G M 2004 Multiple myeloma: a concise review of the disease and treatment options. Online. Available: http://www.myeloma.org 4 Jul 2005
Edwards I., Jones M A, Carr J et al 2004 Clinical reasoning strategies in physical therapy. Physical Therapy 84(4):312–330
Frymoyer J W 1997 The adult spine: principles and practice, 2nd edn. Lippincott-Raven, Philadelphia
Gifford L, Butler D S 1997 The integration of pain sciences into clinical practice. Journal of Hand Therapy 10: 86–95
Greenhalgh S, Selfe J 2003 Malignant myeloma of the spine. Physiotherapy 89(8):486–488 (also available at http://evolve.elsevier.com/Greenhalgh/redflags/)
Greenhalgh S, Selfe J 2004 Margaret: a tragic case of spinal Red Flags and Red Herrings. Physiotherapy 90(2):73–76 (also available at http://evolve.elsevier.com/Greenhalgh/redflags/)
Greenhalgh S, Hollis S, Parnell J, Main C 2005 The reliability of the Linton and Halden initial back pain questionnaire. Manuscript in preparation
Grieve G P 1981 Common vertebral joint problems. Churchill Livingstone, Edinburgh
Hack L M 2004 Invited commentary on: Clinical reasoning strategies in physical therapy. Physical Therapy 84(4):331
Hacker D J 1998 Metacognition in educational theory and practice. Lawrence Erlbaum Associates, London
Hurley D A, Dusoir T E, McDonough S M et al 2001 How effective is the acute low back pain screening

questionnaire for predicting 1 year follow up in patients with low back pain? Clinical Journal of Pain 17(3): 256–263

International Myeloma Foundation 2002 Patient handbook. Edinburgh

Jarvik J G, Deyo R A 2002 Diagnostic evaluation of low back pain with emphasis on imaging. Annals of Internal Medicine 137:586–597

Jones M A 1992 Clinical reasoning in manual therapy. Physical Therapy 72(12):875–884

Jones M A 1995 Clinical reasoning for educators: course notes. Nottingham. Unpublished

Jones M A, Rivett D A 2004 Clinical reasoning for manual therapists. Butterworth Heinemann, Edinburgh

Leventhal E, Crouch M 1997 Are there differences in perceptions of illness across the lifespan? In: Petrie K J, Weinman, J A (eds) Perceptions of health and illness. Harwood Academic Publishers, London

Leventhal H, Benyamini Y, Brownlee S et al 1997 Illness representations. In: Petrie K J, Weinman, J A (eds) Perceptions of health and illness. Harwood Academic Publishers, London

Linton S J 2000 A review of psychological risk factors in back and neck pain. Spine 25(9):1148–1156

MacGregor A J, Andrew T, Sambrook P N, Spector T D 2004 Structural, psychological and genetic influences on low back and neck pain: A study of adult female twins. Arthritis and Rheumatism 51(2):160–167

McKenzie R A, May S 2003a The lumbar spine mechanical diagnosis and therapy, Vol 1. Spinal Publications, Waikanae

McKenzie R A, May S 2003b The lumbar spine mechanical diagnosis and therapy, Vol 2. Spinal publications, Waikanae

Main C, Williams A C C 2002 ABC of psychological medicine: musculoskeletal pain. BMJ 325:534–537
Maltzman J D 2004 Developments in the fight against cancer cachexia. Online. Available: http://www.oncolink.org
Merskey H, Bogduk N 1994 Classification of chronic pain. IASP Press, Seattle
Murphy E A 1997 The logic of medicine, 2nd edn. Johns Hopkins University Press, Baltimore
New Zealand Ministry of Health 2002 Guide to assessing psychosocial yellow flags in acute low back pain. Online. Available: http://www.nzgg.org.nz
NICE 2005 Prevention and treatment of osteoporosis. Online. Available: http://www.nice.org.uk
Richards J S, Nepomuceno C, Riles M, Suer Z 1982 Assessing pain behaviour: the UAB pain behaviour scale. Pain 14:393–398
Roberts L 2000 Flagging the danger signs of low back pain. In: Gifford L (ed) Topical issues in Pain. 2 Biopsychosocial assessment and management, relationships and pain. CNS Press, Falmouth
Round A 2000 Introduction to clinical reasoning. Student BMJ 8:15–17
Schell B B 1998 Clinical reasoning: the basis of practice. In: Neistadt M E, Crepeau E B (eds) Willard and Spackman's Occupational therapy, 9th edn. Lippincott, Philadelphia, p 90–100
Schultz I, Gatchel R J 2005 The handbook of complex occupational disability claims: Early risk identification, intervention and prevention. Kluwer Academic, New York
Scott I 2000 Teaching clinical reasoning a case based approach. In: Jones M A, Higgs J (eds) Clinical reasoning

in the health professions, 2nd edn. Butterworth Heinemann, Oxford
Selfe J 1995 Abnormal illness behaviours in chronic back pain: a practical guide. Journal of Orthopaedic Medicine 17(1):27–28
Spitzer W O 1987 Quebec Task Force report. Spine 12(Suppl 1):S1–S59
Sterling M 2004 A proposed new classification system for whiplash associated disorders – implications for assessment and management. Manual Therapy 9:60–70
Terry P D, Miller A B, Rohan T E 2002 Cigarette smoking and breast cancer: a long latency period. International Journal of Cancer 100(6):723–728
Waddell G 2004 The back pain revolution, 2nd edn. Churchill Livingstone, Edinburgh
Waddell G, McCulloch J A, Kummel E, Venner R M 1980 Nonorganic physical signs in low-back pain. Spine 5(2):117–125
Wardle F M, Maskell A P, Selfe J 2005 Christine: a case of granulocytic sarcoma of the upper trunk of the brachial plexus. Submitted for publication
Wardle F M, Maskell A P, Selfe J 2007 Granulocytic sarcoma – An unusual case of shoulder pain. Journal of the Society of Orthopaedic Medicine 29(1):18–22
WHO 2001 International classification of functioning, disability and health. WHO, Geneva
Wiesel S W, Weinstein J N, Herkowitz H et al 1996, The lumbar spine, International Society for the Study of the Lumbar Spine, 2nd edn. Saunders, Philadelphia
Wilson A 2002 Effective management of musculoskeletal injury. Churchill Livingstone, Edinburgh

Chapter 3

Subjective Examination: Age, Previous Medical History and Lifestyle Questions

CHAPTER CONTENTS

To some readers there may appear to be an imbalance in the content of this book with two chapters devoted to subjective examination and only one to objective examination.

KEY FACT: Deyo et al (1992) argue that the subjective examination provides clinicians with clearer indications of serious pathology than the objective examination.

Further evidence to support the importance of the subjective examination over the objective is found in the CSP research priorities report of 2002 (CSP 2002). In this report the musculoskeletal panel considered the question of physical diagnostic tests commonly used by physiotherapists. They reported that for the assessment of joint dysfunction a wide variety of tests were often described for one structure and that very often these lacked reference to validity and reliability. In addition, a large number of so-called objective tests based on parameters such as range of motion and muscle power relied on subjective clinical statements such 'normal', 'limited' or 'reduced'. Clearly if there are multiple tests with poor validity and reliability there will be problems with interpretation. Therefore relying too heavily on the objective examination for the detection of serious pathology is inappropriate.

During the subjective examination it is the physiotherapist's clinical responsibility to ask the patient questions that are:

- appropriate
- relevant
- sequential
- empathic.

During the subjective examination it is worth remembering the words of Robin McKenzie, who urges clinicians to ask themselves 'Will the answer to the question on the assessment form provide information of practical value in the treatment of this patient?' (McKenzie 1990).

AGE

It is interesting to note, but not surprising, that there are differences in recommendations between various publications regarding the question: At what age does age become a Red Flag?

This is important at both ends of the age spectrum. Should we consider children as small adults complaining of spinal pain or are the pathological processes different? Dillin & Watkins (1992) suggest that, in contrast to adults, in a high proportion of children a specific diagnosis can be determined; however, children may experience considerable delay in receiving a final diagnosis. The diagnosis can be confounded by the fact that intraspinal tumours do not necessarily follow a linear growth pattern, waxing and waning in size, and consequently symptoms can be intermittent (Dillin & Watkins 1992).

A non-specific diagnosis of mechanical back pain is given to 95% of adult back discomfort (CSAG 1994). This is often thought to be a culmination of pathological processes related to degeneration of tissues, including ligament, muscle, disc and bone (Dillin & Watkins 1992), confounded by psychosocial factors (Waddell 2004). These degenerative processes are unlikely to be present in a child.

King (1984) argues that different specific diagnoses could be considered in children under 10 years of age and those 10 years and over. He considers possible causes of back pain in children up to 10 years as:

- infective processes
- tumours of the spinal column or cord.

In children 10 years and over possible causes are:

- spondylolysis/spondylolisthesis
- Scheuermann's disease
- herniated nucleus pulposus
- overuse syndromes
- tumours.

In children and adolescents back pain related to activity and/or worse at night should raise the suspicion of tumour. Dillin & Watkins (1992) consider this particular combination of factors of paramount importance in these age groups with constant back pain.

We have been unable to find a rationale for having a cut-off age of <20 years as a Red Flag. However, this is an age at which rapid physical development has slowed and degenerative processes may have begun. Dillin & Watkins (1992) state that 'our threshold for discovery must be lower for the child than for the adult – the incidence of pathologies is different'.

In the USA and Canada age above 50 years is considered a Red Flag (Bigos 1994, Spitzer 1987). However, in the UK age above 55 years is considered a Red Flag (CSAG 1994). None of these publications gives a clear rationale as to why these particular ages have been selected.

A brief review of the epidemiology of some common cancers may help clinicians understand the importance of age, as the incidence of many cancers increases with age. It is reported (Department of Health 2000) that for some cancers, age may in fact be one of the most useful discriminating factors. People >65 years have 11 times the chance of developing cancer compared to younger people (Goodman et al 1998).

Cancer type and age group (Department of Health 2000, Goodman et al 1998)

- Lung cancer
- Myeloma

  Only 1% or less of cases are diagnosed before 40 years
- Breast cancer

  Only 3–5% of cases are diagnosed before 40 years

  A woman of average life expectancy has a 1 in 9 chance of breast cancer

Cancer type and age group (Department of Health 2000, Goodman et al 1998) – Cont'd

A woman aged 25 years old has a 1 in 21 chance of developing breast cancer

70% of all breast cancer occurs in women aged >50 years

In men aged >60 years familial link is the biggest risk factor

It is usually diagnosed in later stages in older men

- Sarcoma

  Distribution across adult age groups is evenly spread
- Testicular cancer

  Commonest in younger adults <40 years
- Acute leukaemia 2–4 years old
- Neuroblastoma <4 years old
- Bone sarcoma 10–14 years old
- Childhood cancers

Figure 3.1 clearly shows the link between increasing age and increased lung cancer and myeloma. In particular, there is a marked increase between the ages 40–49 and 50–59 and then another even more dramatic increase between the ages 50–59 and 60–69. There would be a high index of suspicion for lung cancer and myeloma in these age groups. However, breast and prostate cancer occur more frequently in the over 65-year-old age group and so have a higher index of suspicion in this group.

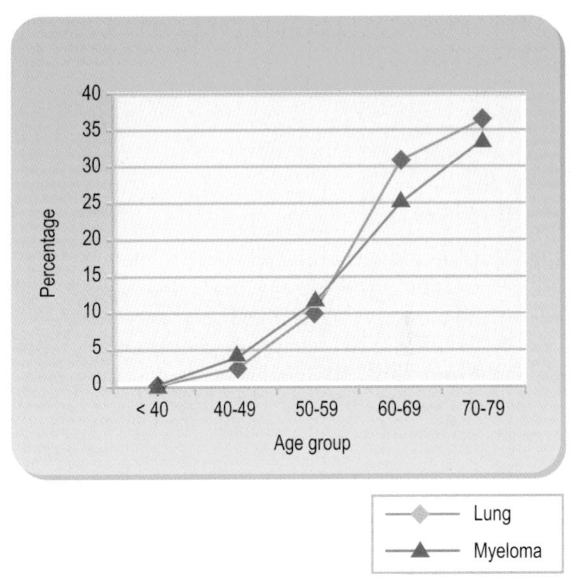

Figure 3.1 Proportions of lung cancer and myeloma cases presenting in different age groups.

In Finland most new cases of breast cancer are found between 50 and 55 years of age (Institute for Statistical and Epidemiological Cancer Research 2004). Seventy per cent of all actual deaths from cancer occur in people over 65 years of age.

Based on the above review rather than focusing on definite cut-off points for age, we would propose the following Red Flag index of suspicion for age:

- <10
- 11–19
- 20–50
- >51

Clinicians should be particularly alert to the possibility of serious pathology presenting in children aged 10 and below and in adults aged 51–65. The ages 11–19 and over 66 should also definitely raise concern but perhaps not to the same level. We would not consider ages 20–50 to require a Red Flag.

MEDICAL HISTORY

A current or past medical history of any of the following conditions should immediately raise serious concerns.

Cancer

For cancer it is usually considered important to establish a personal history. However, we also feel that clinicians should establish whether there has been a family history of cancer, particularly in a first degree relative, i.e. parent/sibling. Positive family history alone would not warrant a referral for a medical opinion; however, it has an important influence on the conditional probability. Therefore adding this information to the list of other concerns the therapist may have strengthens the case for referral (Boissonnault 1995).

The most common warning signs of cancer (Pfalzer 1995)

- Change in bowel or bladder habits
- Sores that do not heal
- Unusual bleeding or discharge
- Thickening or lump in breast or elsewhere
- Indigestion or difficulty swallowing
- Obvious change in wart or mole
- Nagging cough or hoarseness

KEY FACT: Although cancer causes 12% of all deaths worldwide every year (WHO 2004a), it is estimated that neoplastic disease accounts for just 0.7% of all low back pain (Jarvik & Deyo 2002).

The main types of neoplastic disease causing low back pain are:

- multiple myeloma
- metastatic carcinoma
- lymphoma and leukaemia
- spinal cord tumours
- retroperitoneal tumours
- primary vertebral tumours.

Tumours of the spine can remain asymptomatic for long periods of time; symptoms eventually develop for the following reasons (Frymoyer 1997):

- destruction of vertebral cortex and expansion into paravertebral soft tissue
- nerve root compression
- pathological vertebral fracture
- spinal instability
- spinal cord compression.

Intraspinal intrinsic tumours are uncommon; however, extradural tumours are more common, accounting for 22% of primary spinal cord tumours. A classic sign of spinal cord tumours is night pain; bladder dysfunction may also be apparent (Goodman et al 1998).

When considering potential cases of serious pathology, Deyo et al (1992) and Jarvik & Deyo (2002) report that the subjective history is much more useful than the objective physical examination. Table 3.1 shows the estimated accuracy of the history in the diagnosis of cancer in low back pain.

Commonest sources of metastatic cancer (Jarvik & Deyo 2002)

- Breast
- Lung
- Prostate

TABLE 3.1 ESTIMATED ACCURACY OF THE HISTORY IN THE DIAGNOSIS OF CANCER IN LOW BACK PAIN (DEYO & DIEHL 1988)

	Sensitivity	Specificity
Age >50 years	0.77	0.71
Previous history of cancer	0.31	0.98
Unexplained weight loss	0.15	0.94
Failure to improve after 1 month of conservative therapy	0.31	0.90
No relief with bed rest	>0.90	0.46
Duration of pain >1 month	0.50	0.81
Age >50 years + history of cancer + unexplained weight loss + failure to improve after 1 month of conservative therapy	1.00	0.60

According to Rothman & Simeone (1992), patients with a history of breast cancer have an 85% chance of developing bony metastases before death. They also suggest that one of the earliest sites for these metastases is the spine, in particular the thoracic spine. Breast cancer appears in both sexes; 10% of all breast cancer is genetic. Female gender is the biggest risk factor, with less than 1% of breast cancer occurring in men. More than 50% of men have no known risk factors. Men and women whose families have several generations of breast cancer with a BRCA2 mutation on chromosome 13q have the greatest risk. Their risk can be as great as 90%.

Breast cancer in two or more first degree relatives increases the risk by five times. Pregnancy, childbearing and prolonged lactation are considered to have an impact on reducing the risk of breast cancer (Goodman et al 1998).

Many cancers are on the increase; for example, the incidence of multiple myeloma has doubled in the last 10 years and the incidence of non-Hodgkin's lymphoma has doubled since the 1970s.

Multiple myeloma is characterized by an increase in monoclonal plasma cells that leads to abnormally large amounts of a specific immunoglobulin. It is this abnormally large quantity of immunoglobulin that leads to bone pain. Multiple myeloma usually presents gradually but in patients aged over 75 years it is often accompanied by an increased rate of infection. Presymptomatic periods can last between 5 and 20 years; the most frequent initial symptoms are bone pain, particularly back pain (Goodman et al 1998).

Lymphoma describes cancer of the lymphatic system and is divided into two groups:

- Hodgkin's disease – primarily affects young adults
- non-Hodgkin's lymphoma – most commonly presents between 20 and 40 years of age.

The clinical features of Hodgkin's disease include painless swelling of lymph glands in the neck, axilla and groin accompanied by fatigue, fever, night sweats, itching and weight loss; these symptoms are present in 40% of cases. However, asymptomatic enlargement of lymph nodes may be identified on routine examination. Occasionally compression of nerve roots can cause root pain.

In non-Hodgkin's disease lymphadenopathy is generally the first sign, which can develop over months or years. Abdominal lymphoma can cause bloated sensations, gastrointestinal obstruction, bleeding, ascites, leg swelling and back pain. Non-Hodgkin's lymphoma has been reported as presenting as polyarthritis, with fever, night sweats, pallor, fatigue and weight loss. It is important to note that TB, systemic lupus erythematosus, lung and bone cancer can also masquerade as malignant lymphoma (Goodman et al 1998).

A Pancoast tumour, first described by Professor Henry Pancoast in 1924, is an apical tumour in the lung (Gurwood 1999). This pathology must be considered in patients with neck and upper extremity pain accompanied by neurological deficit. Pancoast tumour is rare; less than 5% of lung cancers are Pancoast tumours. Most lung cancer develops lower down in the lungs (Cancer Research UK 2005). The lesion often invades the sympathetic chain and brachial plexus. Typical clinical features include:

- Horner's syndrome:
  - dilation of the pupil

  - ptosis (drooping eyelid)
  - unilateral anhidrosis and flushing of the face
- pain, which can be referred into the shoulder, scapula and along the ulnar nerve distribution of the arm
- wasting of the intrinsic muscles of the hand (Cancer Research UK 2005, Gurwood 1999).

Despite generally being small in size and not readily metastatic, Pancoast tumour has a rapid and almost complete mortality rate (Gurwood 1999).

A commonly asked question amongst physiotherapists is 'How does cancer actually result in death?' According to Maltzman (2004) the most likely cause is as a result of electrolyte imbalance. It is this electrolyte imbalance that results in fatal heart arrhythmias and weakened respiratory muscles leading to pneumonia and fatal systemic infection.

Tuberculosis (TB)

TB infections of the spine are usually 'seeded' from the lungs (Khoo et al 2003). The commonest symptoms are:

- pain in the thoracolumbar junction and decreased range of motion
- weight loss
- fever
- neurological compromise (10–61% of cases)
- malaise
- skeletal involvement (60% in HIV-positive, 1 or 2% in HIV-negative cases)
- abscesses in the groin, trochanteric region or buttock (Leong & Luk 1996).

Although the report of a past medical history of TB should raise an alarm, it is important to remember that following treatment TB can remain dormant for as long as 30–40 years before recurrence (Leong & Luk 1996). It is highly likely that some patients will experience benign back pain unrelated to TB during such a lengthy time period. Therefore it is still very important to think about the conditional probabilities associated with the presence or absence of the other possible symptoms associated with TB. Certainly a past medical history of TB coupled with the report of pain in the thoracolumbar region, which Cyriax (1982) refers to ominously as 'no man's land', should be sufficient evidence to request further investigation.

Spinal tenderness in response to percussion is described by Deyo et al (1992) as having a poor specificity at 0.60 but a sensitivity of 0.86 for bacterial infections. Definitive diagnosis of TB is made by needle biopsy and treatment revolves around an appropriate antimicrobial regimen (Khoo et al 2003), although this is increasingly becoming more challenging with the emergence of drug-resistant strains of TB (WHO 2004b).

HIV/AIDS or injection drug abuse

The human immunodeficiency virus targets CD4+ T cells, a type of white blood cell, which is one of the key cells involved in fighting infection. A healthy immune system has 800–1200 CD4+ T cells per cubic millimetre of blood; once this is reduced to 200 the patient is considered to have AIDS. As the immune system deteriorates it loses its capacity to fight disease and patients become increasingly susceptible to opportunistic illnesses (US Department of Health and Human Services 2004).

How AIDS is spread (US Department of Health and Human Services 2004)

HIV transmission

- Unprotected sex
- Contact with infected blood
- Shared needles or syringes in drug users
- Pregnant women to babies during pregnancy or birth

HIV is not transmitted by

- Sharing food utensils
- Sweat, towels and bedding
- Swimming pools
- Telephones
- Toilet seats, urine, faeces
- Biting insects

HIV is rarely transmitted by

- Needlestick injury

The diagnosis of AIDS, in an HIV-positive patient, requires the presence of at least one of the following opportunistic illnesses:

- pneumonia (present in 21–22% of cases)
- oesophageal candidiasis (present in 13–14.9% of cases)

- TB (present in 21.6% of cases)
- Kaposi's sarcoma (present in 5.5% of cases)
- toxoplasmosis (European Commission 2004, Terence Higgins Trust 2004).

Oesophageal candidiasis is a thrush infection of the oesophagus. The most common symptom is difficulty with swallowing or pain on swallowing, sometimes in association with pain posterior to the sternum. Kaposi's sarcoma was considered rare until the AIDS epidemic; however, it is now much more common, accounting for 10% of all cancers in Kenya and Uganda. Typically it presents as a slow growing pigmented nodule on the leg or foot, although other parts of the body can be affected (Souhami & Tobias 1995). Toxoplasmosis is an infection caused by a parasite called *Toxoplasma gondii*; it can affect all mammals. Between 20% and 50% of the UK population will be infected at some time during their lives. The parasite is found in raw and undercooked meat, infected cat faeces, unwashed, uncooked vegetables and fruit grown in contaminated soil, and unpasteurized goats' milk. A normal immune system keeps the parasite inactive rather than destroying it. Symptoms of the infection are like mild flu in people with healthy immune systems. In patients with HIV/AIDS antibiotic treatment may be required (Terence Higgins Trust 2004).

HIV is frequently spread among injection drug users by sharing needles or syringes contaminated with blood from someone already infected with the virus. In Europe the mean age of problem drug users ranges between 23 years in Ireland and 33 years in Sweden. The majority of drug users who need treatment for health-related problems are men: e.g. Austria 68%; Italy 86% (European Commission 2004).

Osteoporosis

Osteoporosis is recognized internationally as a major healthcare problem. Hip and vertebral fractures are associated with reduced survival as well as considerable morbidity. In the European Union there were an estimated 23.7 million vertebral fractures in 2000. As the population ages, it is predicted that this will rise to 37.3 million in 2050 (European Commission 2004).

However, it is important to note that despite 40 000 vertebral fractures in postmenopausal British women each year, only one third will develop clinical features. Postmenopausal loss of bone mass can be as great as 5% per year due to depletion of hormonal levels. From a clinical perspective it is important to establish when the menopause occurred. It is commonly seen that 10–15 years after menopause fractures start to emerge as a clinical problem.

- 1 in 3 women >65 develop osteoporosis
- 1 in 2 women >70 develop osteoporosis (National Osteoporosis Society 1993).

Although associated with women, it should be remembered that due to the increasing number of elderly people there is now an increased prevalence in both men and women. Osteoporosis can be prevented, it can be treated once it occurs, but it cannot be cured (le Gallez 1998).

Factors contributing to osteoporosis (le Gallez 1998)

Intrinsic

- Sex – women
- Race – whites and Asians
- Family history – increased risk if mother or grandmother had osteoporosis

Extrinsic

- Amenorrhoea
  Eating disorders, oophorectomy, prolonged intense physical activity, late menarche
- Lifestyle
  Smoking (including passive smoking)
  Alcohol >14 units per week female, >21 units per week male
  Poor diet and little exercise
- Drugs
  Corticosteroids. Effects are age- and sex-dependent. An 80-year-old woman with polymyalgia rheumatica taking 10 mg of prednisolone daily could be at a greater risk than a 30-year-old man treated for psoriasis on a dose twice as great.
  Immunosuppressants post transplant surgery.
  Heparin, thyroxine, anticonvulsants, chemotherapy
- Disease
  Chronic inflammatory bowel disease, Crohn's disease
  Kidney, liver disease
  Gastrectomy

LIFESTYLE

Smoking

The scale of the health effects of smoking is vast: 3 out of 10 cancer deaths are smoking related. Smoking kills 13 people every hour in the UK (Secretary of State for Health 1998). Across the European Union half a million people die from the effects of smoking each year. Half of these deaths occur in people aged between 35 and 69, which is well below average life expectancy. Compared to non-smokers, smokers have a poorer diet and higher levels of stress. The most common level of smoking in the European Union in 1995 was between 10 and 14 cigarettes per day (European Commission 2004).

In the UK the smoking epidemic peaked in the 1940s when 2 out of 3 men smoked. The peak for women smokers occurred a little later, post 1948, with 41% of women smoking. In the UK today 26% of adult men and women smoke and 21% of all 15-year-olds smoke (Donnellan 2002). An adolescent who begins smoking at the age of 15 is three times more likely to die of cancer due to smoking than someone who begins in their mid-twenties (Secretary of State for Health 1998). Lung cancer can take twenty years to develop; despite the peak in smoking for women occurring in the late 1940s the rate of mortality in women due to lung cancer is still rising (Donnellan 2002).

Similar to breast cancer, the risk of lung cancer is associated with the quantity smoked and over what period of time the person has smoked for (ASH 2002).

Risk of cancer = Quantity smoked + Length of time smoked

Estimated cause of death for 1000 smokers aged 20 years (Secretary of State for Health 1998)

- 1 murdered
- 6 due to road traffic accident
- 250 in middle age from smoking-related disorders
- 250 in old age from smoking-related disorders

It is also estimated that several hundred non-smokers die each year from lung cancer caused by passive smoking. Although the risk of lung cancer is small from passive smoking, it is 50–100 greater than the risk of lung cancer from exposure to asbestos (Health Education Authority 1991).

There are 4000 chemicals which occur naturally in tobacco, at least 60 of which are carcinogenic (Health Education Authority 1991). With respect to the spine, tobacco smoking adversely affects the circulatory system outside the intervertebral disc, as well as disrupting metabolic processes within the disc.

Effects of smoking on the spine (Nachemson & Vrigard 2000)

- Decreased blood flow
- Decreased nutrition to the disc
- pH of disc lowered
- Mineral content of vertebrae decreased
- Fibrinolytic activity altered
- Increased degenerative changes

Over time these combined processes can lead to degeneration, dehydration, instability and probably low back pain (Rothman & Simeone 1992). In addition, the 'wear and tear' effects of the mechanical stress of coughing which is often associated with smoking need to be considered.

References

ASH 2002 Smoking and cancer; fact sheet 4. Online. Available: http://www.ash.org.uk

Bigos S 1994 Acute low back pain in adults: Clinical practice guideline. US Department of Health and Human Services, Rockville, MD. AHCPR 95-0643

Boissonnault W G 1995 Examination in physical therapy practice: screening for medical disease, 2nd edn. Churchill Livingstone, New York

Cancer Research UK 2005 What is a Pancoast tumour. Online. Available: www.cancerhelp.org.uk 4 Mar 2005

CSAG 1994 Report of a Clinical Standards Advisory Group on Back Pain. HMSO, London

CSP 2002 Priorities for physiotherapy research in the UK: project report. CSP, London

Cyriax J 1982 Textbook of orthopaedic medicine, 8th edn. Baillière Tindall, Eastbourne

Department of Health 2000 Referral guidelines for suspected cancer. London

Deyo R A, Diehl A K 1988 Cancer as a cause of back pain: frequency, clinical presentation and diagnostic strategies. Journal of General and Internal Medicine 3:330–338

Deyo R A, Rainville J, Kent D L 1992 What can the history and physical examination tell us about low back pain? JAMA 268(6):760–765

Dillin W H, Watkins R G 1992 Back pain in children and adolescents. In: Rothman R H, Simeone F A (eds) The spine, 3rd edn. Saunders, Philadelphia, p 231–259

Donnellan C 2002 The smoking debate. Independence, Cambridge

European Commission 2004 Health statistics. Key data on health 2002 (data 1970–2001). European Commission

Frymoyer J W 1997 The adult spine: principles and practice, 2nd edn. Lippincott-Raven, Philadelphia

Goodman C C, Fuller K S, Boissonnault W G 1998 Pathology implications for physical therapists, 2nd edn. Saunders, Philadelphia

Gurwood A S 1999 Horner's syndrome. Optometry Today June: 36–37

Health Education Authority 1991 Passive smoking: Questions and answers. London

Institute for Statistical and Epidemiological Cancer Research 2004 Finnish Cancer Registry. Online. Available: www.cancerregistry.fi

Jarvik J G, Deyo R A 2002 Diagnostic evaluation of low back pain with emphasis on imaging. Annals of Internal Medicine 137:586–597

Khoo L T, Mikawa K, Fessler R G 2003 A surgical revisitation of Pott distemper of the spine. Spine Journal 3:130–145

King H 1984 Back pain in children. Pediatric Clinics of North America 31:1083–1094

le Gallez P 1998 Rheumatology for nurses: patient care. Whurr, London

Leong J C Y, Luk K D K 1996 Spinal infections. In: Wiesel S W et al (eds) The lumbar spine, International Society for the Study of the Lumbar Spine, 2nd edn. Saunders, Philadelphia, p 874–915

McKenzie R A 1990 The cervical and thoracic spine mechanical diagnosis and therapy. Spinal Publications, Waikanae

Maltzman J D 2004 Developments in the fight against cancer cachexia. Online. Available: http://www.oncolink.org

Nachemson A, Vrigard E 2000 Influences of individual factors and smoking on neck and low back pain. In: Nachemson A, Jonsson E (eds) Neck and back pain: The scientific evidence of causes diagnosis and treatment. Lippincott, Williams & Wilkins, Philadelphia

National Osteoporosis Society 1993 Menopause and osteoporosis therapy, practice nurse manual. St Andrews Press, Wells

Pfalzer L A 1995 Oncology: examination, diagnosis and treatment. Medical and surgical considerations. In: Myers R S (ed) Saunders manual of physical therapy practice. Saunders, Philadelphia, p 65

Rothman R H, Simeone F A (eds) 1992 The spine, 3rd edn. Saunders, Philadelphia

Secretary of State for Health 1998 Smoking kills: a White Paper on tobacco. The Stationery Office, London

Souhami R, Tobias J 1995 Cancer and its management, 2nd edn. Blackwell, Oxford
Spitzer W O 1987 Quebec Task Force Report. Spine 12(Suppl 1):S1–S59
Terence Higgins Trust 2004 Toxoplasmosis information for people with HIV and AIDS. London
US Department of Health and Human Services 2004 How HIV causes AIDS. Online. Available: http://www.niaid.nih.gov/factsheets 3 Aug 2004
Waddell G 2004 The back pain revolution, 2nd edn. Churchill Livingstone, Edinburgh
WHO 2004a Cancer. Online. Available: http:www.who.int/cancer 22 Apr 2004
WHO 2004b Tuberculosis infection and transmission. Online. Available: http://www.who.int/mediacentre/factsheets/fs104/en/ 22 Apr 2004

Chapter 4

Subjective Examination: Questions about the Current Episode and Pain

CHAPTER CONTENTS

This chapter continues to emphasize the importance of the subjective examination in detecting serious pathology. The first part of the chapter discusses history of the current episode and pain questions; the second part illustrates an example of a patient–therapist consultation. It takes you on a journey along a theoretical subjective route, highlighting critical cues which affect the clinical decision-making of the physiotherapist. As we have already stated, for clinical reasoning to be successful, the patient and therapist should form an active and balanced partnership in trying to come to an understanding of the patient's condition. The patient scenario provides a practical example of 3D thinking in action. The subjective questioning must consider all aspects of the following warning flags as discussed in Chapters 1 and 2:

- Red
- Yellow
- Blue
- Black
- Orange.

Investigating the behaviour of the patient's pain may help the physiotherapist considerably with differential diagnosis, when faced with a unique clinical scenario. Typically, a change in the location and/or intensity of the symptoms from mechanical musculoskeletal dysfunction can be associated with either an alteration in body posture or specific physical activities. Physiotherapists should be aware of how typical patterns of dysfunction could present (Boissonnault 1995). In simple terms the subjective pain questions should establish:

> *Where was the pain at the beginning, where did it spread or shift to and where is it now?*
>
> (Ombregt et al 2003)

HISTORY OF CURRENT EPISODE QUESTIONS

Weight loss

A frustrating aspect of many publications considering weight loss as a Red Flag is the vague guidance on how much weight loss and over how long should be a cause for concern; for example:

- 'weight loss' (CSAG 1994)
- 'unexplained weight loss' AHCPR report (Bigos 1994)
- 'weight loss' (New Zealand Ministry of Health 2004).

Despite the 10-year period between the CSAG and the New Zealand guidelines no further guidance is given other than 'weight loss' in relation to quantity or time. Only one reference (Boissonnault 1995) was identified that actually quantified weight loss:

> *Unexplained weight change, especially weight loss (5% of body weight over a 4-week period) is a potential symptom of a variety of ailments, including gastrointestinal disorders (e.g., ulcers or cancer), diabetes mellitus, hyperthyroidism, adrenal insufficiency, common infections, malignancies, and depression.*

In addition, few reports actually explain why weight loss may be a Red Flag. Rapid weight loss is usually associated with disseminated tumours rather than small localized tumours (Souhami & Tobias 1995). According to the British Association for Parenteral and Enteral Nutrition (BAPEN) (2003), in the presence of disease, basal metabolic rate increases but physical activity is often decreased and an increase in energy expenditure may not occur. However, there is an increase in protein oxidation and nitrogen loss; therefore in the absence of fluid retention loss of lean body mass occurs.

In later stages of serious pathology cachexic weight loss occurs and is described as drastic loss of body weight of >10%.

Symptoms associated with cachexia (Maltzman 2004)

- Profound loss of appetite
- Lack of sense of taste
- Depressed immune system
- Loss of fat and muscle tissue
- Electrolyte imbalance (leading to weakness, fatigue, pain, paraesthesia and fasciculation)
- Poor outcome of surgery, chemotherapy and radiation therapy
- Unkempt and dishevelled appearance
- Distress associated with changed body image

What clinicians would benefit from is more precise guidance on how much weight loss over what time period they should be concerned about. For example, taller and heavier individuals tend to lose weight faster than those who are shorter and lighter. Hence men tend to lose weight faster than women (BAPEN 2003). Although not designed for this purpose, some guidance may be derived from scales used to assess malnutrition. The Nutrition Risk Score (Reilly et al 1995) uses a scoring system based on absolute weight loss over 3 months (Table 4.1).

However, it should be remembered that absolute weight loss will have differential effects depending on a patient's stature; therefore it may be more useful to consider percentage weight loss.

The Malnutrition Universal Screening Tool (MUST) (BAPEN 2003) uses a scoring system based on

TABLE 4.1 NUTRITION RISK SCORE (REILLY ET AL 1995)

Weight loss in last 3 months (unintentional)	Score
No weight loss	0
0–3 kg weight loss	1
>3–6 kg	2
6 kg or more	3

Cauda equina syndrome

KEY FACT: Although commonly referred to, this is actually a very rare condition with the prevalence among all patients with back pain being estimated at 0.0004 (Jarvik & Deyo 2002).

In the UK it has been estimated that only one case will present annually for every 50 000 patients seen in primary care settings (Office for National Statistics 1995).

The cauda equina consists of spinal nerve roots from L1 distally. Dysfunction of these roots affects motor and sensory function of the pelvic organs, pelvic floor and lower limbs. Cauda equina syndrome is associated with low back pain, unilateral or bilateral leg pain below the knee commonly with segmental neurological deficit, saddle anaesthesia and loss of bladder or bowel function (Tables 4.4 and 4.5). Objective findings may include numbness of the buttocks and perineum usually with widespread sensory disturbance of the legs (Rothman & Simeone 1992). Anal sphincter tone is diminished in 60–80% of cases (Deyo et al 1992). Other important indicators of possible cauda equina syndrome are an extended bladder, confirmed with careful palpation of the lower abdomen, and a patient reporting an inability to pass urine for more than 8 hours (Bartley 2001).

For bladder and bowel to be affected, sacral roots below S2 must be compromised. When sacral nerve roots are injured, the initial response is urinary retention and the bladder becomes flaccid. In a normal bladder a

TABLE 4.4 SENSITIVITY OF SIGNS AND SYMPTOMS OF CAUDA EQUINA SYNDROME (DEYO ET AL 1992)

	Sensitivity
Urinary retention	0.90
Unilateral or bilateral sciatica	>0.80
Sensory motor deficit and reduced straight leg raise	>0.80
Saddle anaesthesia	0.75

sensation of fullness is elicited at 400 mL of fluid. The sensation of the need to void the bowel or bladder is a complex function. Flaccidity of the bladder can result in overflow incontinence possibly associated with inadequate bladder emptying, a rise in residual volume and a reduction in bladder sensitivity (Rothman & Simeone 1992). Sexual dysfunction often accompanies bladder and bowel involvement. This is a very sensitive subject to discuss with a patient. However, Butler (1991) stresses that every sign and symptom should be investigated.

Cauda equina syndrome can present as:

- acute – over 1 week, usually age <40 years, often discal
- chronic – over months or years, usually age >50 years, often stenotic.

TABLE 4.5 SIGNS AND SYMPTOMS OF CAUDA EQUINA SYNDROME IN 45 PATIENTS (NG ET AL 2004)

	Percentage
Perineal numbness	86
Loss of urinary sensation	57
Urinary incontinence	46
Absent anal tone	38
Faecal soiling	15
Painful retention	11
Faecal incontinence	9

Other causes to consider are fracture, malignancy and infection (Rothman & Simeone 1992).

From a physiotherapy perspective the suspicion of cauda equina syndrome should be regarded as an emergency requiring onward specialist referral. However, controversy surrounds the window for the timing of successful decompression, which may be as short as a few hours. Gleave & Macfarlane (2002) suggest that the longer the delay in surgery, the greater the possibility of permanent bladder, bowel, motor and sexual dysfunction. They also suggest that emergency surgery is indicated for patients with an incomplete cauda equina syndrome, but once complete the emergency stage has been missed and delay in surgery at this stage does not detrimentally affect long-term outcome. Cauda equina syndrome occurs in only 1–2% of patients requiring disc surgery.

Systemically unwell – malaise (fever, chills, urinary tract infection)

The presentation of systemic illness varies between children and adults. Children usually present with a short history of systemic illness of several weeks' duration rather than months. In the case of leukaemia, which often presents with back pain, this systemic illness could consist of fever, bruising, pallor, change in mood and fatigue. This short-term systemic presentation can occur in children in many other rare conditions such as:

- juvenile rheumatoid arthritis
- metastatic neuroblastoma
- aplastic anaemia
- idiopathic thrombocytopenia
- infectious mononucleosis (glandular fever).

In contrast, myeloma in adults can remain asymptomatic for years. In early stages myeloma can present with bone pain of varying severity and only vague complaints of tiredness, thirst and nausea (Oken 2002). It is a malignancy affecting plasma cells (Durie 2004). Myeloma results in progressive morbidity by lowering resistance to infection, causing skeletal damage and associated bone pain, hypercalcaemia (one third of patients), anaemia, renal failure and eventually weight loss (Oken 2002). Patients who suffer rapid weight loss and reduced appetite also have associated weakness and fatigue often due to changes in metabolic function such as electrolyte balance (Maltzman 2004). In a small proportion of patients suffering from multiple myeloma, morbidity can also include neuropathy, hyperviscosity of the blood and abnormalities in haemostasis (Durie 2004). Hypercalcaemia causes tiredness, nausea and thirst. High myeloma protein levels can also lead to blood clotting dysfunction, i.e. excessive bruising and bleeding, visual disturbance, headaches, tiredness and ischaemic neurological problems, e.g. carpal tunnel syndrome. The latter is often due to deposition of amyloid Bence Jones proteins (Oken 2002). Neutropenia and hypogammaglobulinaemia raise the possibility of infections, pneumococcal pneumonia being the most common (Durie 2004).

The signs and symptoms of fever have a surprisingly low sensitivity in many cases of spinal infection (Table 4.6).

Raised erythrocyte sedimentation rate (ESR) may occur in a variety of conditions. Table 4.7 shows the normal ranges for ESR in adults. However, a raised ESR is meaningless as an isolated finding. Moreover, some patients with serious pathology will have normal ESR values. This emphasizes that investigations should not be relied on in the first instance and highlights the importance of clinical history-taking and physical examination. In patients with solid tumours an ESR >100 mm

TABLE 4.6 SENSITIVITY OF FEVER (DEYO ET AL 1992)

Diagnosis	Sensitivity
TB, osteomyelitis	0.27
Pyogenic osteomyelitis	0.50
Spinal epidural abscess	0.83

per hour usually suggests metastatic activity (Brigden 1999).

Trauma (fall from height, whiplash, road traffic accident)

Most authorities agree that 'It is surprisingly difficult to damage your spine' and that most people with spinal pain do not actually have any damage to the spine (Roland et al. 1997). An exception to this general rule is cervical spine and whiplash injury or whiplash-associated disorder (WAD). The Quebec Task Force defined whiplash as 'an acceleration–deceleration mechanism of energy transfer to the neck' (Spitzer et al 1995). The amount of energy transfer or force applied to the neck can be very high (Table 4.8) and the time-frame for the flexion/extension acceleration and deceleration is very rapid and is measured in milliseconds.

TABLE 4.7 NORMAL RANGES OF ESR IN ADULTS (BRIGDEN 1999)

Age <50 years	
Men	0–15 mm/hour
Women	0–20 mm/hour
Age >50 years	
Men	0–20 mm/hour
Women	0–30 mm/hour

TABLE 4.8 ESTIMATED FORCES APPLIED TO THE HEAD AND SPINE DURING WHIPLASH INJURY

Authors	Impact speed (km/h)	G-force
Severy et al (1955)	32	12 in extension 16 in flexion
Deng (1989)	63.5	46
McConnell et al (1993)	6–8	4.5

The Quebec Task Force proposed a clinical classification of WAD, which is shown in Table 4.9.

In addition the Quebec Task Force proposed that patients can be classified according to the time elapsed following the injury.

TABLE 4.9 QUEBEC TASK FORCE CLINICAL CLASSIFICATION OF WAD (SPITZER ET AL 1995)

Grade	Clinical presentation
0	No complaint about the neck No physical sign(s)
1	Neck complaint of pain, stiffness or tenderness only No physical sign(s)
2	Neck complaint and Musculoskeletal sign(s) (decreased range of motion and point tenderness)
3	Neck complaint and Neurological sign(s) (decreased or absent deep tendon reflexes, weakness and sensory deficits)
4	Neck complaint and fracture or dislocation Symptoms and disorders that may manifest in all grades include: Deafness Dizziness Tinnitus Headache Memory loss Dysphagia Temporomandibular joint dysfunction

Quebec Task Force patient classification timescales (Spitzer et al 1995)

- Less than 4 days from injury
- 4–21 days from injury
- 22–45 days from injury
- 46–180 days from injury
- In excess of 6 months from injury

Recently the Quebec Task Force clinical classification of WAD has been criticized (Sterling 2004). Sterling argues that grade 2 is too heterogeneous and that psychological dysfunction is not adequately addressed by the classification system. To correct these deficiencies she proposes that grade 2 is subdivided into three categories:

- WAD 2A
- WAD 2B
- WAD 2C.

Interested readers are referred to Sterling (2004) for further details.

A rare but very important symptom occasionally associated with WAD is unilateral neck pain with tongue weakness; this may develop within hours or days of the accident. It is caused by carotid artery dissection, which affects the hypoglossal nerve near to the artery's origin. Ipsilateral Horner's syndrome also sometimes accompanies this problem (Hawkes 2002).

Vertebrobasilar insufficiency (VBI)

The vertebral artery arises from the first part of the subclavian artery. It enters the foramen transversarium of C6 and ascends to C1. After leaving C1 it pierces the dura mater and arachnoid to enter the foramen magnum. Within the skull the two arteries join to form the basilar artery, which in turn leads into the circle of Willis. The vertebral artery is relatively fixed at the foramen magnum and at C2, but between these two points the course of the artery goes through an S bend as it passes behind the lateral mass of the atlas. It is this section of the artery that is subjected to large stretching forces during rotation and is at most risk of injury during inappropriate manual therapy techniques.

VBI produces ischaemia in areas of the brain supplied by the basilar artery: the pons, medulla and cerebellum as well as the central and peripheral vestibular system (Magarey et al 2004). It is therefore not surprising that a wide variety of signs and symptoms can be generated by disruption to the vertebrobasilar circulation (Grant 1994). Dizziness is the most common and is usually the most pronounced symptom of VBI. It is rare for dizziness to occur in isolation; it is usually clustered with other symptoms.

Coman (1986) lists the 5 D's as the most important symptoms associated with VBI. Magarey et al (2004) also highlight the importance of nausea.

5 D's

- Dizziness
- Diplopia
- Drop attacks
- Dysarthria
- Dysphagia

Plus

- Nausea

We would recommend that clinicians explore the 5 D's + 1 during subjective questioning of the patient. There are many other symptoms which have also been reported as associated with VBI (Grant 1994):

- visual perceptual disturbances – spots before the eyes, blurred vision, hallucinations, field defects
- ataxia
- faintness
- light-headedness
- perioral dysaesthesia (tingling around lips)
- nystagmus
- hemianaesthesia.

Similar to whiplash injury there is a large and comprehensive body of literature on the subject of VBI. It is beyond the scope of this pocket guide to discuss this issue in any further detail. Readers are directed to the revised Australian Physiotherapy Association protocol for pre-manipulative testing of the cervical spine as a starting point for this subject (Magarey et al 2004).

Bilateral pins and needles in hands and/or feet

Bilateral pins and needles in the extremities is not a definite indicator of spinal cord dysfunction. It is possible that the patient has a bilateral nerve root compression, bilateral carpal tunnel syndrome or a metabolic condition such as diabetes or thyroid dysfunction. However, pins and needles in all four extremities raises the level of suspicion (Butler 1991).

Patients with spinal cord compression may complain of the following signs and symptoms (Butler 1991):

- a feeling of walking on cotton wool
- loss of dexterity
- diffuse non-specific weakness
- altered sensation
- broad-based jerky gait.

Clinicians should not be reticent about onward referral for a neurological opinion should this be thought necessary.

Previous failed treatment

One of the factors often discussed as a Red Flag is previous failed treatment. This is usually within the context of statements such as 50% of low back pain settles more or less completely within 4 weeks and 90% of low back pain recovers spontaneously within the first 6 weeks (CSAG 1994). McKenzie & May (2003), however, suggest that more recent evidence does not paint such a 'rosy' picture of back pain and that the patient's lifetime experience of back pain is actually one of an intermittent recurring problem, varying in severity, rather than an acute self-limiting one.

It is important to note that failure to respond to treatment is also considered to be a Yellow Flag. As such it becomes apparent that this is a complex issue which is determined by the subtle interaction of a variety of biomedical and psychosocial factors. Briefly, the complexity of previous failed treatment may be compounded by some of the following:

- nature of the condition
- use or non-use of evidence-based practice
- psychosocial issues
- patient–therapist interaction
- patient concordance.

The important point to make here is that unlike patients with mechanical back pain, who have episodic pain which often responds to treatment, patients with serious pathology may initially appear to respond to treatment, but then suffer relapse. It is vital that as well as focusing on the behaviour of specific signs and symptoms during treatment episodes, physiotherapists also monitor the patient's overall health status. This is particularly important when the expected progress as a result of treatment is not being made; vital clues that there may be an underlying serious pathology may be present.

PAIN QUESTIONS

Constant progressive pain

If the patient's pain does not vary with activity or position, the physiotherapist should be suspicious of serious pathology; importantly, as discussed earlier, this may not be true in cases of early serious pathology. During the subjective examination patients will often state that their symptoms are constant. It is essential that in these cases the physiotherapist questions further to identify if the pain 'truly' does not vary at all during a 24-hour period. It is also vitally important to establish how long the pain has behaved in this way. For example, in cases of serious pathology of the spine the initial presentation may be episodic in nature and may also appear to respond to physiotherapy treatment in the early stages (Greenhalgh & Selfe 2003). McKenzie (1990) states that only 30% of patients have truly constant pain. He suggests that many patients get confused when pain has persisted over weeks or months, as pain may be felt intermittently through the day, but some pain is felt every day.

It is of paramount importance that the physiotherapist explores in detail factors that affect the severity of pain. Simple cues for the patient are:

- What makes your pain worse? (aggravating factors)
- Does anything make your pain go away completely? (abolishing factors)
- What makes your pain easier? (easing factors)

Traditionally physiotherapists have tended to consider aggravating and easing factors as being restricted to movement and posture. We suggest a more holistic approach considering, for example, the effects of drug therapy. Current guidelines (CSAG 1994) suggest a role for non-steroidal anti-inflammatories and analgesics in the management of spinal pain. However, patients with established serious pathology will obtain little or no relief from these.

Bickels et al (1999) describe a series of 32 patients with sciatica caused by tumour along the extraspinal course of the sciatic nerve. All patients described insidious onset of pain that progressed, within just one month, to become constant. Twenty-five patients also described significant night pain. Interestingly, more than half the group were able to pinpoint the pain to an exact location which was later found to correspond to the site of the tumour. The authors concluded that ability to locate sciatic pain to an extraspinal point should be considered 'an alarming sign'.

Thoracic pain

Although many patients with benign pathology present with thoracic pain, clinicians need to be alert when faced with this presentation. Patients with mechanical disc disorders of the thoracic spine comprise only 1.96% of patients with mechanical back pain (McKenzie 1990). Thoracic spinal pain is often caused by metastases, most commonly from the lung or breast. Direct venous drainage by the azygos veins from the breast to the circulatory plexus in the thoracic spine accounts for metastatic spread from a primary breast lesion to tumour emboli entering the thoracic region. The emboli pass from the circulatory system to the fertile cancellous bone where they then grow. Lumbar metastases are more commonly prostatic in origin. Once metastases have developed the prognosis is variable. Rapidly progressing neurological symptoms are often associated with poorer outcomes (Wiesel et al 1996). A history of thoracic pain spreading bilaterally and anteriorly should also raise suspicions (Ombregt et al 2003). The commonest symptom of TB is pain in the thoracolumbar junction and decreased range of motion (Khoo et al 2003).

Abdominal pain and changed bowel habits but with no change of medication

Some malignant cancers, for example myeloma, breast and lung, cause hypercalcaemia. It is estimated that approximately 30% of cancer patients will develop hypercalcaemia (Medline Plus 2005).

Hypercalcaemia has already been briefly discussed earlier in the chapter in the 'Systemically unwell' section; some of the symptoms are:

- abdominal pain
- constipation
- nausea and/or vomiting
- poor appetite.

Importantly any change in bowel habits in the absence of a change in medication must be established. The following extract from a case history where the patient was diagnosed with a malignant myeloma illustrates this point.

> *John's problems had begun 10 months previously. His initial symptoms were abdominal pain and increasing problems with constipation despite no changes in medication.* (Greenhalgh & Selfe 2003)

The use of codeine-based analgesics and opioids in cases of spinal pain is common and indeed is indicated in guidelines (CSAG 1994). However, common side effects of these preparations are constipation, nausea and vomiting (BMA 2004).

Severe night pain (disturbed sleep, painkiller consumption)

Investigating symptom behaviour over a 24-hour period includes questions regarding the presence of night pain. However, the physiology behind the phenomenon of night pain is not certain (Frymoyer 1997). Wiesel et al (1996) report that 'Symptoms of back pain at night, pain at rest or a neurological deficit should prompt consideration of a spinal tumour'. However, night pain (pain precluding sleep) has also been associated with mechanical dysfunction as well as the presence of serious pathology, leading to a great deal of confusion and anxiety amongst clinicians.

- Patients with mechanical dysfunction can often provoke pain by turning over in bed; often they simply change position in order to return to sleep.
- Patients with serious pathology often give a history of getting out of bed, pacing, or the need to doze sitting in a chair with an inability to return to sleep.
- Patients with psychological dysfunction often describe disturbed sleep with a pattern of waking in the early hours of the morning.

Concern should be raised if patients report that night pain is the most intense, severe pain episode experienced during a 24-hour period. In contrast, pain associated with mechanical dysfunction is typically most intense and severe during the day when patients are engaged in weight-bearing activities and postures. Exceptions to this general rule are patients who have severe, acute pain for whom even minimal comfort is not achieved in any position (Boissonnault 1995).

Headache

Headaches are common in all age groups (Wilson 2002). According to Cartwright & Godlee (2003), 90% of

Causes of headache (Brier 1999)

- Upper respiratory tract infection
- Depression
- Stress
- Poor posture
- Faulty biomechanics
- Trauma

headaches are tension headaches. Migraine is reported as affecting an estimated 15% of the population (Wilson 2002).

Clinically, Edeling (1988) grades headache by frequency, which she refers to as periodicity (P), and by intensity (I):

P1: pain one day per month or less
P2: pain two or more days per month
P3: pain one or more days per week
P4: pain daily but intermittent
P5: constant pain
I1: mild pain
I2: more than mild pain but tolerable
I3: moderately severe pain
I4: severe pain
I5: intolerable, perhaps suicidal pain.

KEY FACT: It is estimated that only 0.004% of headaches are due to serious pathology (Cartwright & Godlee 2003).

Headaches that increase linearly with unremitting intensity may be consistent with neoplasm. Indicators of serious pathology in headache (Cartwright & Godlee 2003, Hawkes 2002) are:

- sudden onset new severe headache (patients who are not prone to headaches suddenly complain of the first and worst headache in their life; consider vascular tumour or aneurysm)
- progressively worsening headache
- onset of headaches after the age of 50 years
- altered level of consciousness
- recent head or cervical trauma
- abnormal physical findings, especially focal neurology
- meningism
- tender temporal arteries
- cough headache (headache *initiated* by coughing rather than headache aggravated by coughing; approximately 50% will have serious pathology).

As discussed in Chapter 1, differential symptoms of headache due to brain tumour are as follows:

- deep dull constant ache
- aggravated by being upright
- not rhythmic or throbbing
- sometimes severe

- usually relieved by aspirin or cold packs
- does not usually disturb sleep
- aggravated by coughing, sneezing, straining
- nausea not common
- may be associated with cervical dysfunction (Grieve 1994).

EXTRACT FROM A PATIENT–CLINICIAN CONSULTATION

The following extract of a patient subjective examination highlights the Red Flags and the Red Herrings alongside serious pathology clinical reasoning. Other warning flags have been identified for the reader but discussion of these lies outside the remit of this pocket guide.

Key
C = clinician **P** = patient

C Hello Mr X, please come in and sit down. (patient dishevelled, fidgety)

P Thank you.

C My name is Chris. Nice to meet you. We have received a letter from your GP stating . . .

What I would like to do today is to explore the bigger picture of your problem.

When it first developed.

How it has progressed.

What treatment you have had so far and what you are complaining of today.

I will then have a look at you and see what I can find.

We will then talk about my findings and the way forwards.

Is that OK?

P Yes fine. I don't know if I answered those questionnaires OK.

Clinical reasoning

Make the patient feel reassured. Many are nervous of a medical environment. The clinician's body language and tone of voice are important in reassuring and giving confidence from the first patient/client contact to the end of the consultation.

Explain why they are here and what you are going to do in the session so that they know what to expect.

Speak slowly and clearly. There is a lot to take in.

Informed consent.

Linton & Halden (1998) (L&H)
Roland & Morris (1983)

C Yes. They are a great help. Already from these I can see that you are really struggling to keep going and it looks as though you are getting quite low in mood. (Yellow Flag)

Is that right?

P Definitely! (patient constantly moving to gain comfort)

C I will use some of your answers to help me with my questioning. Don't worry, you have done really well.

P Thanks.

C When did you first begin with low back pain ever in your life?

P Oh, I have had it years. I've tried everything. (Yellow Flag)

C Since being a child?

P Oh no. Early 30s.

C And how old are you now?

P 65 years

C Are you retired?

Choose words carefully when discussing and giving feedback on sensitive issues.

It is important to give feedback on completed questionnaires and emphasize their usefulness.

The L&H can be used to direct the subjective questions.

Even those with chronic pain can develop serious pathology. The full subjective history gives a complete picture.

Could there be any pars defects due to exercise leading to spondylolisthesis?

P Yes. I retired 15 years ago. Early retirement.

C Was that because of your health?

P Yes.

C Was it your back?

P Yes but I also have problems with depression. I was in hospital for a while. (Yellow and Orange Flags)

C So do you have incapacity or disability benefits now?

P No I have had a bit of trouble with benefit reviews recently. I have had my benefits withdrawn, I did get a job in an office but I have been off sick for some time; in fact my boss is putting me under pressure to go back. (Yellow, Blue and Black Flags)

C OK. How did your low back pain first start?

P It started when I worked in the abattoir. I twisted and lifted a carcass onto a high table and I felt my back 'go'. I knew that I had done something. (🐟?)

They did not care about Health & Safety then. (Yellow Flag)

Clinical reasoning

Any infection in past?
(brucellosis, see Ch. 1)

Not likely now as 30–35 years later (conditional probability).

C Could you continue working?

P No. I had to go home and went to bed. The doctor came out and told me to go to bed for 2 weeks so I did.

C Was it better then?

P No, I had to have physio. That helped a bit. I went back to work but I have had problems on and off ever since. But for the last 3 years it has been constant.

C Do these episodes usually settle on their own?

P Sometimes I have needed physio, I still try to do my exercises. I have seen an osteopath once or twice. I have had acupuncture and seen a chiropractor. It is difficult to get to see these people. There are long waits and it costs a fortune. (Yellow Flag)

C Did any of them help?

P Yes. Usually it got better but this time it is different.

C OK – Tell me about how this episode started?

P It is all in my buttocks and it comes into my stomach

Clinical reasoning

Up to this point it could very well be chronic pain. Remember three-dimensional thinking adds: verbal and non-verbal communication.

C When did this episode start?

P Ages ago.

C 2–3 months?

P Oh longer than that. 6 months I would say.

C How did it begin?

P I woke up with it. I had been helping the wife move some furniture a few days before. I put it down to that bloody wardrobe. (Yellow Flag)

C Did you feel anything at the time?

P No – but I had not done anything else that may have caused it

C OK – so what exactly did you feel?

P Well, I had been a bit off colour for a few months. I started with pains in my stomach and constipation. I have seen the consultant at the hospital.

I went in for a day. I had some investigations but everything was OK.

C What did you have?

Clinical reasoning

Try to get the patient to stick to a chronological order. Be courteous in bringing them back to the order of progression of symptoms or your clinical reasoning may become confused.

P Endosc . . . Can't remember what it was called. I had the camera . . . but he said everything was OK.

C Good. Are those symptoms any better?

P No, I am on some tablets for it.

This is what I take (hands list to clinician) but they don't work.

C Thank you, that is really helpful. Had you changed your diet or tablets when the constipation occurred?

P No.

C So these don't help.

P No and now I have this backache as well.

C Do you have any leg pain?

P No, not really, it aches a bit in my thighs but my legs feel really weak

C Any pins and needles or numbness?

P Sometimes my feet feel a bit funny.

C Where?

Clinical reasoning

Do not be over-reliant on other clinicians' diagnosis or negative investigation findings. Trust your own 3D thinking as conditions can and do change.

P All over.

C Big toe and inside of your foot right across to the outside of the foot and little toe?

P Yes. Sometimes my feet don't feel right.

C Both feet – have you been tested for diabetes?

P Yes and I have not got it.

C OK. Is that pins and needles getting worse or better or the same?

P Difficult to say, I think it is getting worse, the pain certainly is.

C What makes your pain feel worse?

P Everything really, I can't stand for long. I can only walk from here to the grocers (50 metres). I can't sit for long. For the last 2 weeks I have slept in a chair.

C Do you sleep?

P I doze on and off.

C What happens if you go to bed?

Clinical reasoning

Consider differential diagnosis

P It became so bad trying to lie down – it was better to stay in the chair.

C Do you sleep during the day?

P No, I can't sleep.

C What makes it feel better?

P Nothing really – I try a hot water bottle but even the tramadol does not help. I have tried loads of pills that the doctor gave me but it does not seem to help.

C Are your bladder and bowels OK?

P Well, I suffer with constipation still.

C Do you feel that this is related to your tablets or is that normal for you?

P Oh no, I used to be OK. This began before the backache – before I started the tablets – it just happened. That is one of the reasons that I saw the doctor at the hospital – but he said everything is OK. He said that you would sort me out.

C (Smile) – OK.

C Have you lost any weight.

P Yes, I can't eat – the pain – I have no appetite.

C How much have you lost?

P Well I was 64 kg but when they weighed me at the hospital I was 56 kg.

C How long have you been losing weight?

P Difficult to say. I'm not sure – about 6–8 weeks.

C Right (said positively). Do you feel well?

P No, I'm tired, can't sleep, sick of the pain, I feel sick, no, I don't feel well.

C Do you smoke?

P No.

C Have you ever?

P Oh yes. I used to until this started.

C OK. How many did you smoke?

P About 20–25 on a bad day.

C When did you start smoking?

Clinical reasoning

The index of suspicion suggests this may be a problem but need to know time period.

Clearly this is a major problem.

Don't leave the questioning on smoking there.

EU average 1995 = 10–14 per day

P Oh when I was a lad – 16 years, about 15 or 16.

C What about medical history? Have you had any serious illnesses or operations other than you have told me? There does not appear to be anything else in the notes.

P No . . . No I don't think so.

C OK – what about your family – parents, brothers, sisters. Did they have anything significant in their medical history?

P No, eh well my dad died of a heart attack. My mum had cancer.

C Which sort – do you know?

P Breast cancer.

C What about brothers, sisters, grandparents?

P I don't know about my grandparents and I haven't seen my sister for years. She lives abroad – we lost touch.

If I hadn't lifted that bloody wardrobe.

C That is all the questions for now. Well done. What I am going to do now is have a look at you.

Clinical reasoning

If sister or grandparents did have breast cancer – much higher risk (see Ch. 2).

In this scenario we have tried to illustrate how the patient's response directs the physiotherapist's questioning and how the physiotherapist asks questions that conform to the guidelines we introduced at the beginning of Chapter 3, i.e. they are:

- appropriate
- relevant
- sequential
- empathic.

Throughout the scenario we have also highlighted the warning flags as they arise as this helps to show how the direction of questioning can be influenced. This reinforces the points made about clinical reasoning and 3D thinking in Chapter 2. We argued that for successful clinical reasoning to occur an active partnership between the patient and the physiotherapist needs to be formed in order to come to an understanding of the patient's condition. Unfortunately in many scenarios a paternalistic relationship develops where the therapist becomes dominant whilst the patient is relegated to a passive role. When this type of relationship develops it is unlikely to produce a satisfactory result.

In the scenario the following warning signs were found:

- 30
- 7 Yellow Flags
- 1 Blue Flag
- 1 Black Flag

- 1 Orange Flag
- 4 🐟.

Clearly a large volume of information has been gained from the subjective examination, a lot of which, in this case, is highly suggestive of serious pathology. Using the wealth of valuable information gained from the subjective examination, the physiotherapist must now decide which objective tests are appropriate for the individual patient. It is important that the physiotherapist 'mentally pauses/takes stock' at this point to assimilate the large volume of verbal and non-verbal information they have gathered. This will give them the opportunity to see 'the wood from the trees' so that they can carefully plan the objective examination. Patients with potentially serious pathology and in obvious distress will need to be examined quite differently from those with minor mechanical problems. Planning which tests need to be conducted, before actually starting the objective examination, is vital. This avoids wasting the patient's and physiotherapist's time by completing irrelevant tests that will yield little additional information and perhaps more importantly avoids unnecessarily subjecting patients to uncomfortable procedures.

References

Bartley R 2001 Nerve root compression and cauda equina syndrome. In: Bartley R, Coffey P (eds) Management of low back pain in primary care. Butterworth Heinemann, Oxford, p 63–67

Bickels J, Kahanovitz N, Rubert C K 1999 Extraspinal bone and soft-tissue tumours as a cause of sciatica. Spine 24(15):1611–1616

Bigos S 1994 Acute low back pain in adults: Clinical practice guideline. US Department of Health and Human Services, Rockville, MD. AHCPR 95-0643

BMA 2004 BNF, 48th edn. BMA and BPS, London

Boissonnault W G 1995 Examination in physical therapy practice: screening for medical disease, 2nd edn. Churchill Livingstone, New York

Brier S R 1999 Primary care orthopaedics. Mosby, St Louis

Brigden M L 1999 Clinical utility of the erythrocyte sedimentation rate. American Journal of Family Physicians 60:1443–1450

British Association for Parenteral and Enteral Nutrition (BAPEN) 2003 Malnutrition Universal Screening Tool (MUST). Redditch

Butler D S 1991 Mobilisation of the nervous system. Churchill Livingstone, Melbourne

Cartwright S, Godlee C 2003 Churchill's pocket book of general practice, 2nd edn. Churchill Livingstone, Edinburgh

Coman W 1986 Dizziness related to ENT conditions. In: Grieve G P (ed) Modern manual therapy of the vertebral column. Churchill Livingstone, Edinburgh, p 303–324

CSAG 1994 Report of a Clinical Standards Advisory Group on Back Pain. HMSO, London

Deng Y C 1989 Anthropometric dummy neck modeling and injury considerations, Accident Prevention 21: 85–100

Deyo R A, Rainville J, Kent D L 1992 What can the history and physical examination tell us about low back pain? JAMA 268(6):760–765

Durie B G M 2004 Multiple myeloma: a concise review of the disease and treatment options. http://www.myeloma.org 4 Jul 2005

Edeling J 1988 Manual therapy for chronic headache. Butterworths, London

Frymoyer J W 1997 The adult spine: principles and practice, 2nd edn. Lippincott-Raven, Philadelphia

Gleave J R W, Macfarlane R 2002 Cauda equina syndrome: what is the relationship between timing of surgery and outcome? British Journal of Neurosurgery 16(4):325–328

Grant R 1994 Vertebral artery insufficiency: a clinical protocol for premanipulative testing of the cervical spine. In: Boyling J D, Palastanga N (eds) Grieve's modern manual therapy, 2nd edn. Churchill Livingstone, Edinburgh, p 371–380

Greenhalgh S, Selfe J 2003 Malignant myeloma of the spine. Physiotherapy 89(8):486–488 (also available at http://evolve.elsevier.com/Greenhalgh/redflags/)

Grieve G P 1994 The masqueraders. In: Boyling J D, Palastanga N (eds) Grieve's modern manual therapy: the vertebral column, 2nd edn. Churchill Livingstone, Edinburgh, p 841–856

Hawkes C 2002 Smart handles and red flags in neurological diagnosis. Hospital Medicine 63(12):732–742

Jarvik J G, Deyo R A 2002 Diagnostic evaluation of low back pain with emphasis on imaging. Annals of Internal Medicine 137:586–597

Khoo L T, Mikawa K, Fessler R G 2003 A surgical revisitation of Pott distemper of the spine. Spine Journal 3:130–145

Linton S J, Halden K 1998 Can we screen for problematic back pain? A screening questionnaire for predicting outcome in acute and sub-acute back pain. Clinical Journal of Pain 14:200–215

McConnell W E, Howard P R, Guzman H M 1993 Analysis of human test subject responses to low velocity rear end impacts. Society for Automotive Engineers, Detroit, SP-975

McKenzie R A 1990 The cervical and thoracic spine: mechanical diagnosis and therapy. Spinal Publications, Waikanae

McKenzie R A, May S 2003 The lumbar spine: mechanical diagnosis and therapy, Vol 1. Spinal Publications, Waikanae

Magarey M E, Rebbeck T, Coughlan B et al 2004 Pre-manipulative testing of the cervical spine: review, revision and new clinical guidelines. Manual Therapy 9:95–108

Maltzman J D 2004 Developments in the fight against cancer cachexia. Online. Available: http://www.oncolink.org

Medline Plus 2005 Hypercalcaemia. Online. Available: http://www.nlm.nih.gov/medlineplus

New Zealand Ministry of Health 2004 New Zealand Acute Low Back Pain Guidelines. Online. Available: http://www.nzgg.org.nz 4 Apr 2005

Ng L C L, Tafazal S, Longworth S, Sell P 2004 Cauda equina syndrome: an audit. Can we do better? Journal of Orthopaedic Medicine 26(2):98–101

Office for National Statistics 1995, Morbidity statistics from general practice: 4th national study 1991–1992. HMSO, London

Oken M M 2002 Management of myeloma: current and future approaches. Online. Available http://www.moffitt.usf.edu\pubs\ccj\v5n3\article2

Ombregt L, Bisschop P, ter Veer H J 2003 A system of orthopaedic medicine, 2nd edn. Churchill Livingstone, London

Reilly H M, Martineau J K, Moran A, Kennedy H 1995 Nutritional screening evaluation and implementation of a simple nutrition risk score, Clinical Nutrition 14:269–273

Roland M O, Morris R W 1983 A study of the natural history of back pain. Part 1: Development of a reliable and sensitive measure of disability in low back pain. Spine 8:141–144

Roland M, Waddell G, Klaber-Moffett J et al 1997 The back book, 3rd edn. The Stationery Office, Norwich

Rothman R H, Simeone F A (eds) 1992 The spine, 3rd edn. Saunders, Philadelphia

Severy D M, Mathewson J H, Bechtol C O 1955 Controlled automobile rear end collisions and investigation of related engineering and medical phenomena. Canadian Services Medical Journal 11:727–759

Souhami R, Tobias J 1995 Cancer and its management, 2nd edn. Blackwell, Oxford

Spitzer W O, Skovron H L, Salmi L R et al 1995 Scientific monograph of the Quebec Task Force on whiplash-associated disorders. Spine 20:7S–73S

Sterling M 2004 A proposed new classification system for whiplash associated disorders – implications for assessment and management. Manual Therapy 9:60–70

Wiesel S W, Weinstein J N, Herkowitz H et al 1996 The lumbar spine, International Society for the Study of the Lumbar Spine, 2nd edn. Saunders, Philadelphia

Wilson A 2002 Effective management of musculoskeletal injury. Churchill Livingstone, Edinburgh

Chapter **5**

Objective Examination

CHAPTER CONTENTS

For the purpose of this chapter the objective tests considered will be confined to the neuromusculoskeletal assessment of the spine and limbs. Extended scope examinations of the abdomen, for example, will not be discussed. As we have discussed in Chapter 2, the objective examination begins with the therapist's observation and interpretation of initial cues from the patient when they first meet, even before any verbal communication takes place. The examination should be performed in a logical order with minimal disruption to patient comfort by avoiding unnecessary changes in patient position. The objective assessment may even need to be adapted and carried out in a chair or sitting on the side of the bed if the level of pain is so severe that lying is not possible.

All examinations of the spinal column should, where possible, consider the following:

- general physical appearance
- deformity
- deviation
- muscle spasm
- paravertebral mass
- pattern of neurological deficit
- cord compression.

PHYSICAL APPEARANCE

Looks unwell

It is surprising how many publications suggest that clinicians assess whether the patient looks unwell; yet most do not provide any guidance or suggestions about what an unwell person looks like. This is interesting as there is a large element of subjectivity involved in this type of judgement and many patients who are seriously ill can 'look quite healthy' in the early stages.

One of the publications that does give more specific guidance is Cyriax (1982), who states 'Inspection of the patient's face may help to decide how disabling his pain has been; severe pain leading to sleepless nights shows on the patient's face.' The following extract from a case history of a patient with a malignant myeloma also helps to illustrate how physical appearance can alert the clinician to potentially serious pathology: 'He appeared unwell with a sallow complexion, slightly dishevelled appearance and poorly fitting clothes' (Greenhalgh & Selfe 2003).

General signs that the patient may be unwell

- Pallor/flushing
- Sweating
- Altered complexion; sallow/jaundiced
- Tremor/shaking
- Tired/drawn
- Dishevelled/unkempt
- Halitosis
- Poorly fitting clothes.

These signs may be explained by the complex metabolic changes that occur with serious pathology. In particular, electrolyte imbalance, hypercalcaemia and weight loss can cause a number of these signs.

Spinal deformity

The key clinical features of interest are spinal deformity with marked spinal muscle spasm and unexpectedly severe limitation of movement. It is important to identify deformities that are rapidly reversible as these may be associated with benign mechanical syndromes. A rapid onset of scoliosis (deviation) can be also be associated with osteoid osteoma or osteoblastoma. This deformity may not appear while the patient is standing upright but may present on forward flexion. The concave side of the deformity is usually on the same side as the tumour. Frymoyer (1997) suggests the tumour is often at the apex of the curve.

Mass

Often tumours cannot be seen or felt. However, should a mass be identified size, location, mobility and tenderness are key clinical features. Bickels et al (1999), in a series of 32 patients with sciatic nerve tumours, reported that 13 patients had a palpable mass. Recent changes in the structure must also be established. In some cases, swelling is one of the first presenting signs. With some tumours, e.g. osteosarcoma, the overlying skin may be warm (Goodman et al 1998).

INABILITY TO LIE SUPINE

Although not necessarily restricted to night time, inability to lie supine is listed as a Red Flag in a number of clinical guidelines (Bigos 1994, New Zealand Ministry of Health 2004). Frymoyer (1997) reports that the pain symptoms associated with inability to lie supine are probably due to increased pressure on the affected segment. This is illustrated clinically by 'John now complained of constant unremitting pain, was unable to sleep and had not been to bed for a couple of months; he dozed in a chair' (Greenhalgh & Selfe 2003), and by 'sleeping upright in a chair helped' (Greenhalgh & Selfe 2004).

BIZARRE NEUROLOGICAL DEFICIT

According to Wiesel et al (1996), the formal style of neurological examination practised today developed in the 19th century. An early pioneer of this field was Leasague, who first described the straight leg raise (SLR) test in 1880. Later Henry Head contributed significantly to the understanding of dermatomes by observation of patients with herpes zoster.

Frymoyer (1997) reports that in cases of serious pathology neurological deficit is rarely the first symptom; despite this observation, in those with serious spinal pathology:

- 70% will have neurological deficit by the time of diagnosis
- 50% of those with spinal cord compression will develop symptoms of the compression before diagnosis is made.

The presence of gross multiple neurological deficit is usually obvious. More subtle expansion of neurological deficit can be more difficult to identify. In the cervical spine, due to the angle of the emerging nerve root in proximity to the disc, segmental neurological deficit is usually clearly defined. In contrast, in the lumbar spine neurological deficit can present a more confusing picture. As the nerve root angle is more vertical, a bulging disc causing nerve entrapment can result in a less clearly defined segmental deficit, as one disc bulge could appear to compromise one or two nerve roots; however, this can still be within normal segmental limits.

As thorough a neurological examination as possible (this is dictated by the severity of the patient's pain) must always be carried out if neural compressive or destructive disorders are indicated from the subjective history. Neurological examination for the thoracic spine is often overlooked, but it is as important as that for lumbar and/or cervical spines and may need to be included. The presence of neurological deficit and thoracic pain should prompt the physiotherapist to consider the possibility of malignancy, infection or fracture. Positive answers to the following questions should be considered with a relatively high index of suspicion.

- Is more than one root affected?
- Are there more than two roots affected?
- Are there more than three roots affected?
- Are there any cord signs?

The following neurological findings during a spinal examination also need to be considered with a relatively high index of suspicion:

- C1–C2: Paraesthesia, occipitoparietal region. Weakness rare.
- C3: No myotomal involvement, cutaneous analgesia uncommon.
- C4: Anaesthesia in horizontal band along spine of scapula, mid-deltoid and clavicle.
- C8: alone Pancoast tumour.
- T1: Weakness in the intrinsic muscles of the hand, paraesthesia and cutaneous analgesia in ulnar aspect of hand: consider pulmonary tumour, Pancoast tumour or vertebral metastases.
- T2: Dermatomal numbness, neurological deficit rare.
- L1/L2 root signs (often associated with lung cancer, malignancy in the vertebrae or upper femur).

It is interesting to note from the list above that in general within each spinal region the most cephalad vertebral segments, i.e. C1/2, T1/2 and L1/2, appear to have a greater predisposition to serious pathology than the more caudal segments. This phenomenon appears to be a subtle addition to Grieve's observation that the more cephalad the serious pathology the poorer the prognosis (Grieve 1981).

Lhermitte's sign is provoked by cervical flexion; it consists of an electric shock like feeling which shoots down the spine and occasionally into the arms.

KEY FACT: Lhermitte's sign is almost pathognomonic of multiple sclerosis.

Rarely, it also occurs in cervical spondylosis and cervical spinal cord tumours. A reversed Lhermitte's sign is provoked by cervical extension; this is strongly associated with cervical spondylosis. However, it is important to note that very infrequently patients with multiple sclerosis also complain of a positive reversed Lhermitte's sign (Hawkes 2002).

MARKED PARTIAL ARTICULAR RESTRICTION OF MOVEMENT

Deviation on movement is often associated with mechanical dysfunction; it could present following a disc derangement or it could be caused by soft tissue shortening after trauma. Deviation on movement may also be associated with neurological deficit. However, Goodman et al (1998) warn that these signs could also be present in the case of tumours. It is the first author's experience that the most common movement restriction presenting in the presence of serious pathology, in the lumbar spine, is a marked restriction of flexion.

LOSS OF SPHINCTER TONE AND ALTERED S4 SENSATION

As previously stated in Chapter 4, disturbances of normal bladder and bowel control are rare, serious neurological symptoms that require thorough investigation. The sphincter of the bladder and musculature controlling the rectum are supplied by S3, S4 and S5. These nerve roots also supply sensation to the saddle area, a round area between the upper buttocks and above the anus.

If cauda equina syndrome is suspected a rectal examination must be performed by an appropriate clinician, in a timely manner. A normal rectal reflex would be a sudden contraction of the anal sphincter on light touch (Wiesel et al 1996). Saddle sensory disturbance can be tested either by light touch or by pin-prick. We would recommend that in any case where the subjective history suggests S4 sensation abnormalities the sensory disturbance should be tested. Testing can be carried out with the patient in either side lying or crook lying, depending on the patient's level of discomfort.

SPASM

Muscle spasm is synonymous with low back pain and is always due to an underlying cause. Its clinical significance, however, is poorly defined. Occasionally the muscle contraction is so severe unilaterally that a deviation or scoliosis can occur. The correlation between muscle spasm, pain and other objective clinical measures is poorly supported by a strong evidence base. However, Ombregt et al (2003) suggest that muscle spasm precluding movement should always be considered suspicious.

VERTEBRAL ARTERY TESTING

Whilst pre-manipulative protocols have been very clear, in terms of specific testing routines, there is some question over the appropriateness of routine clinical testing of the vertebral artery. The difficulty lies in the fact that vertebral artery testing itself is a procedure associated with some risk (Table 5.1). Therefore there is a real danger that the clinician may in fact be placing the patient at unnecessary risk by performing inappropriate vertebral artery testing.

Magarey et al (2004) have published a revised set of clinical guidelines for the testing of the vertebral artery. These new clinical guidelines are less rigid and prescriptive than the previous format of the APA (Australian Physiotherapy Association) pre-manipulative

TABLE 5.1 SAFETY OF VERTEBRAL ARTERY TESTING

Authors	Conclusions
Refshauge & Gass (1995)	Testing must be performed with extreme caution to avoid exacerbating potentially serious pathology
Grant (1994)	The test procedures themselves hold certain risks
Meadows (1992)	The testing procedure itself might provoke the very occlusion that the therapist is attempting to avoid

testing protocol. This is to allow clinicians a greater degree of autonomy in practice and places much more emphasis on clinical reasoning. These new guidelines also place a much greater degree of emphasis on the importance of detecting potential indicators of risk during the patient subjective examination. This reflects the fact that current research evidence is inconclusive as to which are the most valid vertebral artery screening tests, and that provocation testing is potentially harmful.

As adverse incidents involving the vertebral artery seem to be associated with cervical rotation, sustained end range rotation is the only mandatory test included in these new guidelines. Any additional testing should be guided by clinical reasoning appropriate to the individual patient.

Mandatory pre-manipulative vertebral artery testing (Magarey et al 2004)

- Sustained end range rotation in supine or sitting

UPPER CERVICAL INSTABILITY TESTS

These tests are sometimes used after whiplash injury; great care should be taken in performing any upper cervical stability tests. We would recommend that full training in both the application and the interpretation of the tests should be undertaken before attempting these tests on a patient, as they are potentially harmful.

Subjective findings that may suggest cervical instability

- Occipital numbness or paraesthesia
- Headaches
- Vertigo
- Tinnitus
- Visual disturbances

Petty & Moore (2001) describe the following upper cervical stress tests:

- distraction test
- posterior stability test of the atlanto-occipital joint
- anterior stability test of the atlanto-occipital joint
- Sharp–Purser test
- anterior translation stress test of the atlas on the axis
- lateral stability stress test for the atlanto-axial joint
- lateral flexion stress test for the alar ligaments
- rotational stress test for the alar ligament.

The tests are considered positive if the patient reports one or more of the following:

- loss of balance in relation to head movement
- unilateral pain along the length of the tongue
- paraesthesia in face or lip
- bilateral or quadrilateral limb paraesthesia
- nystagmus.

POSITIVE EXTENSOR PLANTAR RESPONSE

According to Gifford (2000) this test was first described by Babinski in 1896.

KEY FACT: This test should be included in any spinal examination irrespective of level of spine affected.

There is often confusion as to why this test should be included in the examination of cervical and thoracic lesions; however, as it is used as a tool to identify upper motor neuron lesions and the spinal cord ends at L1, its inclusion in the examination of cervical and thoracic lesions would appear self-evident.

The plantar reflex is usually tested using a sharp object such as the sharp end of a tendon hammer. The sharp object is stroked from the heel, along the lateral aspect of the foot to the base of the fifth metatarsal progressing the sweep medially to the base of the big toe.

- A normal response is flexion of the toes.
- An abnormal response is a slow extension of the great toe with spreading of the adjacent toes (Ombregt et al 2003).

In small reflex reactions it can be helpful to observe the great toe. In some extreme cases an abnormal reaction can be accompanied by hip and knee flexion. This abnormal response must not be confused with the patient's reaction due to foot sensitivity.

Hawkes (2002) warns that if an easily obtained abnormal plantar response is elicited, multiple sclerosis (MS) should be considered. However, he goes on to suggest that the interpretation of the sign can be controversial so clinicians need to take care. If a patient reports unilateral symptoms but presents with a bilateral abnormal plantar response, this can also indicate MS. In these cases the patient will often complain of a unilateral heavy or numb leg with a completely normal other leg. The reason for this presentation is the presence of a number of plaques only some of which will give rise to symptoms

DISTURBED GAIT

Generalized upper and lower extremity weakness with associated gait disturbance could suggest myelopathy. The initial presentation of myelopathy can include neck pain, numb, cold or painful hands and a reduction in fine finger movements followed by proprioceptive changes and a subtle broad-based gait. The presence of clonus on sustained dorsiflexion of the foot can also be indicative of myelopathy (Frymoyer 1997).

Cervical myelopathy can occur as a consequence of cervical spondylosis. Gait disturbance is often the issue that raises concern. Classical neurological features include lower motor lesions at the level of the lesion and upper motor neuron lesions below. Early myelopathy can masquerade as bilateral carpal tunnel syndrome, with patients complaining of paraesthesia and problems with dexterity (Frymoyer 1997).

SUMMARY

As we have already stated earlier, all examinations of the spinal column should consider the following:

- general physical appearance
- deformity
- deviation
- muscle spasm
- paravertebral mass
- pattern of neurological deficit
- cord compression.

With respect to specific spinal regions, Table 5.2 gives other indicators of serious spinal pathology and their possible interpretation.

The Red Flags are only given as a guide to help the physiotherapist in the clinical decision-making process. However, the skill of the practitioner with these objective tests and their interpretation strengthens with experience. No two clinical presentations are exactly the same but clinical reasoning is based on information collected from a number of different sources in each individual patient presentation (Gifford & Butler 1997). Further investigations may be necessary to confirm or clarify the clinical picture, but must not replace the clinical examination. Similarly investigation findings must not be considered in isolation without

TABLE 5.2 INDICATORS OF SERIOUS SPINAL PATHOLOGY AND THEIR POSSIBLE INTERPRETATION (FRYMOYER 1997, OMBREGT ET AL 2003, WIESEL ET AL 1996)

Patient position	Test/Action/Movement/Sign	Possible interpretation
Lumbar spine		
Standing	Persistent severe restriction of flexion Side flexion away: only painful movement Marked articular signs and absent dural signs Gross limitation of both side flexions	Non-specific serious pathology
Supine	Sacroiliac joint Hip joint Sign of the buttock	Consider osteomyelitis, neoplasm of ilium or upper femoral head, fractured sacrum
Supine	Warm foot	Non-specific serious pathology

Thoracic spine		
Standing	T1 stretch	Non-specific serious pathology
Standing	Side flexion away: only painful movement Full articular pattern Severe restriction of extension Flexion with rigid thoracic segment	Pulmonary or abdominal tumour Non-specific serious pathology
Standing	A difference of less than 4.5 cm between full inspiration and full expiration	Ankylosing spondylitis
Sitting	Plantar reflex – positive plantar response	Upper motor neuron lesion
Supine/prone	Dermatomal numbness	Non-specific serious pathology

table continues

TABLE 5.2 INDICATORS OF SERIOUS SPINAL PATHOLOGY AND THEIR POSSIBLE INTERPRETATION (FRYMOYER 1997, OMBREGT ET AL 2003, WIESEL ET AL 1996) — Cont'd

Patient position	Test/Action/Movement/Sign	Possible interpretation
Cervical spine		
Standing	Side flexion away from pain: only painful movement	Possible fracture or metastases of scapula, lesion in clavicle, ribs or apex of lung
	Resisted cervical movements – weakness	Consider vertebral metastases, fractured rib, spinous process of C7 or T1, wedge fracture vertebral body, glandular fever, post-concussional syndrome, retropharyngeal abscess

the additional data from the subjective and objective examination.

References

Bickels J, Kahanovitz N, Rubert C K et al 1999 Extraspinal bone and soft-tissue tumours as a cause of sciatica. Spine 24(15):1611–1616

Bigos S 1994 Acute low back pain in adults: Clinical practice guideline, US Department of Health and Human Services. Rockville, MD. AHCPR 95-0643

Cyriax J 1982 Textbook of orthopaedic medicine, 8th edn. Baillière Tindall, Eastbourne

Frymoyer J W 1997 The adult spine: principles and practice, 2nd edn. Lippincott-Raven, Philadelphia

Gifford L 2000, Topical issues in pain 2. CNS Press, Falmouth

Gifford L, Butler D S 1997 The integration of pain sciences into clinical practice. Journal of Hand Therapy 10:86–95

Goodman C C, Fuller K S, Boissonnault W G 1998 Pathology implications for physical therapists, 2nd edn. Saunders, Philadelphia

Grant R 1994 Physical therapy of the cervical and thoracic spine. Churchill Livingstone, New York

Greenhalgh S, Selfe J 2003 Malignant myeloma of the spine. Physiotherapy 89(8):486–488 (also available at http://evolve.elsevier.com/Greenhalgh/redflags/)

Greenhalgh S, Selfe J 2004 Margaret: a tragic case of spinal Red Flags and Red Herrings, Physiotherapy 90(2):73–76 (also available at http://evolve.elsevier.com/Greenhalgh/redflags/)

Grieve G P 1981 Common vertebral joint problems. Churchill Livingstone, Edinburgh

Hawkes C 2002 Smart handles and red flags in neurological diagnosis. Hospital Medicine 63(12):732–742

Magarey M E, Rebbeck T, Coughlan B et al 2004 Pre-manipulative testing of the cervical spine: review, revision and new clinical guidelines. Manual Therapy 9:95–108

Meadows J 1992 Safety considerations in vertebral artery testing. IFOMT 5th International Conference, Vail, CO

New Zealand Ministry of Health 2004 New Zealand Acute Low Back Pain Guidelines. Online. Available http://www.nzgg.org.nz 4 Apr 2005

Ombregt L, Bisschop P, ter Veer H J 2003 A system of orthopaedic medicine, 2nd edn. Churchill Livingstone, London

Petty N, Moore A P 2001 Neuromusculoskeletal examination and assessment, 2nd edn. Churchill Livingstone, Edinburgh

Refshauge K, Gass E 1995 Musculoskeletal physiotherapy. Clinical science and practice. Butterworth-Heinemann, Oxford

Wiesel S W, Weinstein J N, Herkowitz H et al 1996 The lumbar spine, International Society for the Study of the Lumbar Spine, 2nd edn. Saunders, Philadelphia

Chapter **6**

Conclusion

CHAPTER CONTENTS

HIERARCHICAL LIST OF RED FLAGS

(Note: This list is also available to download at http://evolve.elsevier.com/Greenhalgh/redflags/)

- Age >50 years + history of cancer + unexplained weight loss + failure to improve after 1 month of conservative therapy

- Age <10 or >51
- Medical history (current or past) of
  - Cancer
  - TB
  - HIV/AIDS or injection drug abuse
  - Osteoporosis
- Weight loss >10% body weight (3–6 months)
- Cauda equina syndrome
- Severe night pain
- Loss of sphincter tone and altered S4 sensation
- Positive extensor plantar response

- Age 11–19
- Weight loss 5–10% body weight (3–6 months)
- Constant progressive pain
- Abdominal pain and changed bowel habits but with no change of medication
- Inability to lie supine
- Bizarre neurological deficit

- Spasm
- Disturbed gait
- Steroids

- Weight loss <5% body weight (3–6 months)
- Smoking
- Systemically unwell
- Trauma
- Vertebrobasilar insufficiency
- Bilateral pins and needles in hands and/or feet
- Previous failed treatment
- Thoracic pain
- Headache
- Physical appearance
- Marked partial articular restriction of movement
- Vertebral artery testing
- Upper cervical instability tests

RED FLAGS NOT RED HERRINGS – THE CLINICIAN'S PERSPECTIVE

One of the questions we have been asked while writing this book is:

> *What do I do once I have found a number of Red Flags and am suspicious that this patient has a serious spinal pathology?*

Although a plethora of guidelines exist in relation to the management of low back pain, all literature about suspected serious pathology advises the same thing:

- **Refer for *early* specialist opinion.**

The CSAG (1994) guidelines suggest:

Urgent referral for specialist investigation, generally to an orthopaedic surgeon or rheumatologist; depending on local availability.

The Arthritis and Musculoskeletal Alliance (ARMA 2004) recommend:

People in whom serious disease is suspected should be referred without delay to specialist services for investigation and treatment in accordance with National Guidelines, such as NICE referral protocols.

The Prodigy (2005) guidelines recommend:

Consider prompt investigation or specialist referral (less than 4 weeks) for anyone with a red flag for possible spinal pathology.

The route to this early specialist opinion will be peculiar to each medical subculture. The key to successfully managing these serious cases is to have a robust, well-established pathway in place to access, once these patients present (Fig. 6.1). Whether the patient is identified in primary care, secondary care or the private sector, the pathway needs to be understood; indeed, a well-established pathway may already be in place. If there is no developed route it is important that stakeholders communicate and work together to develop a fast, effective patient journey, enhancing optimum outcome. This pathway is as important as a thorough

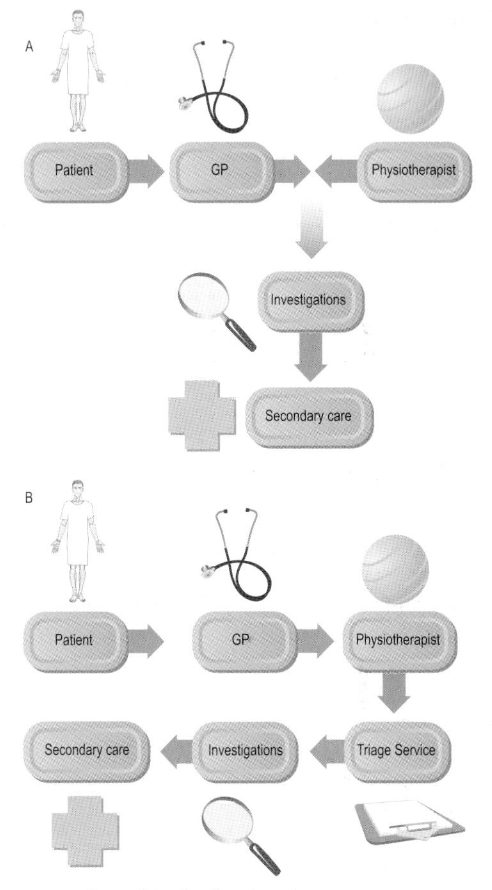

Figure 6.1 Examples of referral pathways.

subjective and objective assessment. Consideration of how these serious cases will be managed can enhance early detection and appropriate intervention, which can have a huge impact on the patient's medical management and final outcome. Although these cases account for only 1% of spinal cases, pattern recognition of that clinical experience is profound and the memory will often remain with the clinician for some time. Both the patient and the clinician deserve the best support possible; consider how familiar you are with your local pathway before you need to use it.

Investigations may include a combination of some of the following:

- X-ray
- magnetic resonance scan
- computer tomography
- bone scan.

Although many readers of this pocket guide will not be responsible for organizing complex investigations, those who are should consider the following questions before proceeding:

- Why do I order these tests?
- What am I going to look for in the result?
- If I find it, will it affect my diagnosis?
- How will this affect my management of the case?
- Will this ultimately benefit the patient? (Asher 1954)

Ordering unnecessary investigations not only wastes valuable resources but can also cause unnecessary anxiety and distress for patients and their families. If in doubt it is recommended that clinicians discuss individual cases with a radiologist who will be able to advise on the most appropriate test.

Sensitive, empathic communication is essential with any patient. Remember good eye contact and body language, use listening skills carefully (the patient gives good clues to the condition in their general conversation). Reassure appropriately and do not create unnecessary anxiety. Be prepared for the question: 'Do you think that something is seriously wrong with me?'

Phrases such as: 'I think that we need to look into your problem a little further so that we can see more clearly what is going on. We need to make absolutely sure that you are given the best and most appropriate treatment' are particularly useful.

These phrases create much less anxiety than phrases indicating a large element of doubt or phrases expressing alarm or inappropriate concern, such as: 'I think there may be something seriously wrong that is causing your pain. I think we need to get you seen by a specialist as soon as possible.'

On the other hand, do not give unrealistic reassurance – 'I am 100% sure that there is nothing seriously wrong with you' – when there is some doubt in your mind.

Do not be afraid to suggest: 'You are obviously really struggling, physiotherapy is not appropriate at this stage but we do need to find out exactly what might be causing it. I am going to . . .

Explain carefully to the patient the next step on your particular pathway and give the patient and carer time to ask any questions. Do not guess or bluff, as this can easily be picked up by the patient and confidence in the clinician lost. However, be emotionally intelligent with your answers.

Do not forget that the purpose of this book is to enable the physiotherapist to identify patients who have a high index of suspicion for serious spinal pathology and then alert the appropriate authorities. It is not encouraging clinicians to attempt to diagnose these cases. In addition, it was never the intention of the authors to cause the reader to over-focus on serious spinal pathology, consequently putting most patients in a 'possible serious pathology' box. It attempts to give further tools to equip physiotherapists in their three-dimensional thinking process and clinical reasoning.

Finally, to equip the physiotherapist in accordance with the principles advocated by the NHS Modernisation Agency, we would suggest the following care bundle. This is an evidence-based, simple list of key steps to equip the physiotherapist to identify serious pathology of the spine.

Care bundle

- Diagnostic triage
- Biopsychosocial approach
- Red Flags
- Red Herrings
- Patient referral pathway for serious pathology

References

ARMA 2004 Standards of care for people with low back pain. Online. Available: www.arma.uk.net
Asher R 1954 Straight and crooked thinking. BMJ September: 460–462
CSAG 1994 Report of a Clinical Standards Advisory Group on Back Pain. HMSO, London
Prodigy 2005 Low back pain. Online. Available: www.prodigy.nhs.uk/guidance

Index

Please note that page references to any non-textual information in boxes are in *italic* print